SENSATION IN THE NIGHT

Waking Up To Breast Cancer

What You Still Don't Know

Susan Armenti

Note to Reader:

The ideas, suggestions and procedures in this book are in no way to be a substitute for professional medical advice and consulting with your physician(s). All matters regarding your health require expert professional medical supervision. The publisher and author take no responsibility or liability for any loss, damage or injury allegedly resulting from following any information, suggestions or ideas in this book. Each individual is responsible for their own medical case and needs to seek out and follow professional medical advice. The author is not a doctor but just a patient explaining what happened to her and others she knows who have had a breast cancer diagnosis. This is a work of non-fiction however some names and details have been altered. No parts of this book are to be duplicated without the permission of the author.

www.sensationinthenight.com

Illustrations on pages 7,31
by George Retseck.
Illustration on page 207
printed with the permission of Dr. Karl Breuing.
Cover photo from Corbis.
ISBN-10: 0615665357
EAN-13: 9780615665351
Creative Thoroughbred

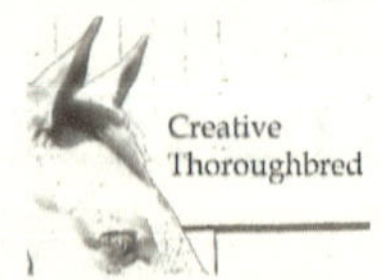

To my parents, Pat and Fred, who gave me everything I needed.
And to Cinder, who was there for every word.
And to anyone who has yet to tell.

Table of Contents

Foreword

Cancer is a small six-letter word with a complex meaning and far-reaching consequences. It is often unpredictable and unforgiving. Even the strongest of us commonly fall apart if given the diagnosis of cancer. For a woman, hearing the words, "I'm sorry, but you have breast cancer," changes her life forever.

This is a very personal story about my only sister, Susan, and her struggle with breast cancer. In it she openly expresses her fears and feelings around dealing with this medical monster that often strikes without cause or warning. As she navigated through the complex maze of medical jargon, misinformation and impersonal situations, she also learned what is right and what is wrong with our health care system. She learned about her disease by sifting through countless books and articles to chart her course in fighting this illness. Unfortunately, she did much of this alone, not wanting to burden others with her problem. She even kept this secret from me, her older brother, for nearly seven years. Regrettably, her story is not unique. It is played out daily by thousands of people who have been diagnosed with cancer. Over the years, women in particular have been stigmatized by cancer resulting in emotions of shame and despair over an initial diagnosis of breast cancer. And for Susan, the fewer people that knew, the less grave she could make of the circumstances.

The medical field has advanced almost beyond comprehension. The amount of new procedures, drugs, devices and regulations makes it nearly humanly impossible to be a generalist anymore. As it has become more complex, it has also become more specialized. Doctors and nurses usually feel comfortable discussing their own particular area of expertise but may not be so knowledgeable outside their narrow scope of practice. The numerous office visits a patient endures usually result in patients only getting pieces of information which they then have to assemble themselves to get a complete picture of what is happening in their lives. Susan had this same experience and tells of her frustration in dealing with the system: a health care system which is far from perfect in which expert opinions often conflict and even misinformation is disseminated by well-intentioned caregivers. How is a lay person to know the difference between right and wrong?

Beyond the technical aspects of medicine, Susan also talks about the personal encounters that shaped her attitude towards her cancer. She was never interested in medicine as a child and actually had a real aversion to hospitals. I clearly remember her protesting to my parents if she was forced to accompany the rest of the family to see a sick friend or relative in the hospital. But due to this chapter in her life she was forced to live life in a hospital for more days than she would like to remember. And like anyone in "foreign territory" she was ultra-alert to her surroundings. Not much, if anything, went unnoticed. The result has been her learning as much as possible about her illness and with it I think a renewed appreciation for life and a purpose that would not have been possible without having endured the struggle. Her purpose in writing this book is to help others who find themselves in a similar situation.

I'm very proud of my sister for having the courage to chronicle her ordeal and put down on paper the very private aspects of her life in the wish that others may have an easier time dealing with breast cancer. I hope that the reader of this book heeds Susan's advice to ask the tough questions and challenge the medical opinions put forth by the "experts." If you are armed with the knowledge and understanding Susan has gained through her research and personal experience, you too can ask those difficult questions.

I've learned over the years that most patients know their own bodies and sense when something is wrong. With the information in this book you no longer need to feel totally alone and helpless. The knowledge and information Susan shares will give you the confidence to seek out the best and most appropriate medical treatment should the day ever come when you are told, "I'm sorry, but you have breast cancer."

Her loving brother,
Fred

Frederick R. Armenti, M.D.
Attending Cardiothoracic Surgeon
Chairman, Department of Surgery
Chairman, Multidisciplinary Thoracic Oncology Conference
McLaren Regional Medical Center
Flint, Michigan

Introduction

To confront cancer is to encounter a parallel species, one perhaps more adaptable to survival then even we are.

–Siddhartha Mukherjee, *The Emperor of All Maladies*

There is nothing quite like a cancer diagnosis to stop the forward motion of your life. This book exists only because I wanted *you* to know what I didn't when all this started for me 16 years ago. For as much as doctors are there to facilitate wellness, healing comes from the patient.

Experience 'has taught me breast cancer is a battle with the most uncertain of outcomes. Entering into battle you have needs you never before thought much about. You must accumulate equipment, certain information, advisors, courage and fellow soldiers. This book is meant to arm you with some of what you need as you fight. And I don't take that word lightly. It is a *fight*.

The statistics will likely shock you – and rightly so. *One in eight American women will be diagnosed with breast cancer in her lifetime.* Approximately 39,520 women and 450 men died of breast cancer in 2011 in the U.S. – equivalent to the number of deaths from the 9/11 tragedy times 13 and then some. This is not a single event but one that happens every year, year after year in the United States. And globally breast cancer deaths are on the rise as well.

In America in 2011 an estimated 230,480 new cases of female invasive breast cancer were diagnosed plus as an estimated 57,650 additional cases of in situ breast cancer, according to the American

Cancer Society. Breast cancer is the leading cause of death for women between the ages of 40 and 55. And around the world in 2010 there were 1.5 million new breast cancer cases diagnosed. Most women, high risk or not, contemplate at some point, *Will I get breast cancer?*

Yet perhaps the statistic that fuels the fear and speaks to the unknown is this: according to the National Breast Cancer Coalition an estimated 3 million women have breast cancer or a history of breast cancer in America but as many as 1 million of them don't know it yet.

While the numbers are staggering, for me it all comes down to one woman. The woman who just found out she has breast cancer; the one who is crying in her car or her office over the news. I've done both so I know it happens. And in light of the controversial 2009 USPS Task Force's "mammography guidelines," my story where early monitoring and pushing for a correct diagnosis may have saved my life is perhaps the best counter-balance to, in my opinion, these misleading and dangerous recommendations.

Intuition leads me here. Had I relied solely on medical advice from the medical experts, my story may have been very different – and not in a good way. I have heard too many stories of misdiagnosis and experienced it myself not to sound the alarm; not to do so seems irresponsible. Misdiagnosis happens and it happens often enough that you need to be aware of it.

My purpose is two-fold. To increase awareness for screening and for women to listen to their own internal voice. More than the current information would have you think, it is incumbent on the individual woman to monitor her own health, heed the warning signs, if there are any, and continually get screening mammograms and additional tests if needed. While mammograms are far from perfect, especially in younger women, they are still the best screening device we have. Apart from that, to dismiss your inner voice, your instinct, your internal wisdom without fully investigating if there is anything physically wrong can be a costly mistake. According to Dr. Susan Love's *Breast Book*, "80% of breast cancers that are *not* found on a mammogram are discovered by the woman herself."

While many associate cancer with pain I want to make it clear that without detection this disease grows silently, most often painlessly, in its early stages. If you wait to feel bad physically or see physical signs, the disease has often progressed to a dangerous level. Since early detection is the best defense, women's awareness of their own bodies cannot be underestimated. My hope is to offer insight into what you need to look out for and what to ask if something suspicious is discovered. Ignoring the possibility of breast cancer does not make the risk go away. And we are all at risk – some more than others.

Others have been public about the shock of a breast cancer diagnosis – Betty Rollins, Betty Ford, Olivia Newton-John, Carly Simon, Suzanne Sommers, Sheryl Crow, Melissa Etheridge, Lynn Redgrave, Elizabeth Edwards, Christina Applegate – to name a few, and their voices are memorable due to their celebrity. But I am not a celebrity. I'm simply a woman trying to make sense of all this information (and much of it is conflicting) in order to retain my life. Breast cancer treatment can be full of choices: lumpectomy vs. mastectomy, mammogram vs. MRI, radiation/chemotherapy before or after surgery, if at all, and on and on. The options and therefore the decisions are daunting.

It took some time for me to be public about my diagnosis. For the first seven years of dealing with breast cancer, my boyfriend at the time, Michael, was the only person, other than my medical caretakers, who knew what was going on with me medically. Since I didn't go through readily apparent treatments at first, I had this option. I have since explained the diagnosis and the results of my treatment with friends and family. When I broke the news seven years later some of my family and many of my friends couldn't understand my need for privacy, and to this day I am sure some are still hurt by my reluctance to share it with them right from the beginning. I hope they understand it wasn't about them. It was about me. Both my parents died of cancer. I lived through what a cancer diagnosis does to the entire conversation. It consumes it. I wasn't going to allow that if I could prevent it.

As the years passed I decided what I went through could make a positive difference for someone else. I believe if I can share my story, and the stories of some of the women I have met along the way, it will hopefully be useful to someone newly diagnosed or someone who has reached another crossroad in her treatment or even someone sharing the journey: a friend, a mate, an adult child, a mother, a father, a sister. Or, *most importantly*, someone who "feels" something abnormal is going on in her breasts and hasn't obtained medical confirmation of her intuition or suspicion. I want to support her investigation.

Women being private and remaining silent about breast cancer had a long-standing tradition. For the record, it has been only a couple of decades since cancer, breast cancer included, has been discussed openly. Thanks to women like Betty Ford and Betty Rollins, organizations like the Susan G. Komen Foundation and doctors like Susan Love, M.D., it has come out of the shadows. But it is true that many breast cancer patients still keep their diagnosis quiet due to a feeling of shame or fear of repercussions like job loss. Or they may have a desire to keep it to themselves if that is possible.

I didn't want to "become the disease" and yet it would have been comforting to find someone who had been through it and could tell me her experience. For anyone who has yet to tell others, I dedicate this to you. It can be a difficult and lonely decision (some would say courageous, others would say unwise) but it was the right one for me at the time and it may be the right one for you. The point being, it is up to *you*. I know there is a loud and pushy voice about "gathering support" but you don't owe anyone an explanation or "the truth" about your health. It is your right to keep it private, and although it may not be the easiest decision, it is your right to make it.

My intention and hope is that men will read this book too. Primarily so they will know that not only are they not immune from getting breast cancer – men get breast cancer and in numbers far greater than most would guess – but because I want them to have an understanding of what the women in their lives are facing. If you are a partner, father, brother, son or a male friend my sincere hope is you will read this so that you are not stumbling around in the dark and retreating. We need your focus, your caretaking, your humor and your desire to make it better for us. You won't be able to cure us but you are more instrumental in our coping and healing than you can imagine.

A writer begins with a point of view and mine is as a patient. Believe me, I wished at times I could do my own biopsies, my own surgeries and write my own prescriptions for medicines. But I am not a doctor. I was always the patient: the one waiting for treatment, answers, help, a different diagnosis, results, a warm blanket, pain medicine, news of some breakthrough development like a blood test that will tell you if this will return, not just confirm it when it has returned.

Sixteen years have passed and not much has changed. Many in the medical community will tell you how things have progressed – they no longer always remove all your lymph nodes, breast-conserving surgery is more prevalent, there are anti-nausea drugs that are more effective. All those things, while good, aren't good enough. Frankly, I'm still waiting. I'm still waiting for a way to accurately predict, prevent and eradicate cancer.

And, with a most hopeful heart, I have written this with the professional caretaking community in mind. I remember when my dad was at Jefferson Hospital in Philadelphia during his final days in 1993, for treatment of leukemia. Nurses would come in and prick his skin every hour for blood. On this one particular day a nurse came in and stabbed his finger far more violently than necessary. Blood spurted out. He was really good-natured but on this day he said, "Hey, show some mercy." She looked at him perplexed; it seemed a routine enough act to her. I'll say it here in case you need to hear it. When you have cancer very little is routine, so if you are a caretaker, "show some mercy," please.

As I was writing I did a lot of meditating on my intention of service, my motivation surrounding this book. After meditating I wrote in my journal:

"I don't want you to be alone. I will be your sister, your aunt, your mother. I will only be two-dimensional and unable to leave the page but I am here in black and white, whenever you need me. I'm going to tell you the truth, or as much of it as I know. I see how scared you are and it is completely understandable. I know you see the fear and sadness in the faces of the people who love you. Don't blame them, they are hurting too. They can't help it. You will only get through this one minute at a time. My only real advice is to stay as present as you can. The past has left and the future has yet to arrive but right here you are alive and can feel it all. Be grateful that you can feel and ask for pain medicine when you feel too much. You are brave to walk this way – never forget that." 12/15/07

In February of 2008, a few months after that journal entry, my 22-year-old niece, Amanda, was diagnosed with a pareosteal-osteosarcoma in her left leg. Her mom had passed away four years earlier and it was clear to me that she needed me to be there. Some of my first words to her were, "You aren't going to go through this alone." So in March 2008 I spent a month in Boston at Massachusetts General Hospital taking care of her. Maybe these earlier words were meant for her, maybe they have a broader meaning, I don't know. But that month of "hospital life" just reinforced my belief that having a patient advocate while hospitalized is essential. It is my deepest hope you ask for and get the support you need.

Part 1

1

My Story

Our girl is in trouble.

– Aurora Greenway played by
Shirley MacLaine in the film *Terms Of Endearment*

A sensation in the night... That is what it was for me, my first encounter with breast cancer. The year was 1996 and I was 41 years old. I was in the dark, literally. At three o'clock in the morning, my left breast woke me up. Not with a pain, but a sensation that I had never experienced before. It wasn't that full feeling you get when you have your period; this was clearly different.

"Activity" is how I described it to my boyfriend, Michael. We were in bed, I turned on the light and I woke him up. "I think something is going on in there." Rubbing my left breast, the area right over my heart, I felt something deep inside.

"What? What do you feel?" he asked while he looked at my breasts like so many other nights. I'm sure they looked the same to him: big, round, warm 34Ds. I've always had great breasts. How could something so good be suddenly bad?

"I don't know, it just feels like it's...busy in there." Confused about how to describe the sensation I was feeling.

"You're lumpy," he reminded me. He was right. I am lumpy and have always had dense and lumpy breasts. But did I intuit something else?

That night, as soon as I was conscious of the feeling, it went away. Wide awake I was no longer in such a receptive state and I was not able to sense the "activity." I finally went back to sleep. However, when it woke me up again the next night, I decided I needed to see someone about it.

TIP: If you sense abnormal activity, check it out even if you can't feel a lump. Trust your instincts and intuition. They are there for good reasons. We have insulated ourselves from an instinctual response to so many things. We medicate our sleep, our moods and our symptoms and sometimes that is necessary. But our species' instinctual responses are survival mechanisms and we need to acknowledge them, understand them and use them to our advantage. Early detection is our best defense against breast cancer.

My breasts have always been somewhat of a mystery to me and have kept me guessing my whole adult life. I had my first mammogram at 18 because there seemed to be something suspicious in my right breast close to my arm. I had been having regular mammograms and been told how "dense" my breasts were ever since that first one, in 1973. Around the year 2000 a technician told me that because of this density my mammograms were "hard to read." I had never heard that before. This is now common knowledge – that young women often have dense breasts and their mammograms are notoriously hard to read – but prior to hearing that in 2000 I thought what you see is what you get and had full faith in mammography's ability to pinpoint a potential problem.

TIP: If you are young (under 40) and feel something isn't right and a mammogram doesn't show anything,

insist on another test: an ultrasound, or maybe an MRI. If an abnormality is found, then a needle or core biopsy can be done. Your breast tissue may be so dense that the mammogram is not able to detect a problem; but getting a "negative" does not mean you are in the clear.

Up until 1996 my mammograms had always come back fine but I had never been woken up in the middle of the night before by a "sensation in my breast" – this was highly unusual. I took my latest mammogram films and went to see Dr. Jerrold Steiner at Cedars-Sinai Medical Center, in Los Angeles.

He examined me and said, "Yes, you are lumpy," not telling me anything I didn't already know. I showed him the spot that I thought was "acting up" and there seemed to be some fibroid tissue in that area so he said he would biopsy the area with a fine needle aspiration (FNA) to remove some cells and see if anything was going on.

As I was leaving his office, Dr. Steiner said to reassure me, "I'm not worried about you. I'll have the results in a couple of days and I'll call you."

I walked out of there thinking, "Well, that's a relief. Someone who knows something about breast cancer said he isn't worried about me so I won't worry either," and I waited for the results. A couple days later, Dr. Steiner phoned. "Susan, there are abnormal cells in the biopsy." Much to the surprise of both of us, the slides showed abnormal cells and he recommended an "open biopsy" of the site. I panicked. "What? But I thought I was fine?"

TIP: A biopsy is a way for doctors to tell if what appears to be suspicious is a problem. Every biopsy is not necessarily harmless, as you are changing the architecture of the breast and later this could make it more difficult to detect a real problem. However, you sometimes don't know for certain until you put in a needle, so it is often necessary. Of course

unless they get the right spot they aren't always accurate. If you find yourself on this road you will realize it is a balancing act of risks and procedures, the road ahead not always a clear path.

When Dr. Steiner told me I needed an "open biopsy" or "lumpectomy" I wasn't ready for the news. Is anyone ever ready? I would need anesthesia and he would surgically remove the area in question along with some surrounding tissue. The goal would be to have nothing but healthy tissue left, and "clear margins." But as there was no lump that you could feel, I thought, "Is this really necessary?"

I decided I needed a second opinion so I went to a cancer center, City of Hope, in Duarte, California, to Dr. Lawrence Wagman. Dr. Wagman explained that I had another option, a core biopsy which, as he described it, sounded less invasive than an open biopsy or lumpectomy. So in September of 1996 at City of Hope, I had a core biopsy. While a core biopsy is less invasive, it is in fact a diagnostic procedure, not meant as a therapy. During the procedure I lay on a table while a radiologist, whom I don't think was very experienced or skilled (I don't know which) used a gun-like device and shot a metal cylinder into my breast while reading an ultrasound. The "gun" is loud, like a cap gun, and the cylinder it sends into the breast retrieves a tissue sample. Due to the "blasting nature" and repeated sampling I am suspect as to the core's innocent reputation but it does not require surgery, which is certainly a benefit. It was very painful. My boyfriend, Michael, who was in the room with me, mirrored my distress, jumping when the gun went off : it was that loud. Seven times the radiologist "shot me" and a half an hour later the procedure was over. I know now they didn't give me enough lidocaine and didn't allow enough time for it to numb me.

TIP: If you have a core biopsy make sure they give you

plenty of local anesthetic, which in my case was lidocaine. You should be numb and while you may feel pressure there is absolutely no need to feel sharp pain. If you feel any pain, stop, and make them wait for what they have administered to take effect before they resume the procedure or make them give you more pain medicine. Don't let them rush you.

The diagnosis came back "benign fibroadenoma" – a non-cancerous mass. The assumption was that this type of biopsy was more substantial and conclusive than the FNA so of course, when it came back benign, I wanted to believe, and the doctors concurred, nothing was wrong. Hey, I did my part. I checked it out and look, I'm fine. Right?

1997

In 1997 I had a routine mammogram. Nothing suspicious showed up. The area in question was thicker, and often drew my attention but with so much scar tissue from the biopsies I didn't find that so surprising. My biggest problem that year was a sad break up with Michael, the only person with whom I had shared what I had gone through medically. It certainly made the break up that much harder. I was really alone with this now. It was the same August weekend that Princess Diana died. I moved back to my own house and tried to put it all behind me.

1998-1999

Valentine's weekend I got a black and white cocker spaniel puppy. I had to say goodbye to my boyfriend's dog, Cello, when we split up even though he had always followed me around the house (the dog not the boyfriend). A cancer scare puts things in perspective. I love animals and decided I wasn't going to live without a dog. She was the cutest dog ever and the best decision I ever made. I called her Cinder and she has been my constant companion ever since. You spend a lot of time home in bed recovering and having a four-legged friend who offers unconditional acceptance and love helps.

In 1998 I had another mammogram at City of Hope and "micro calcifications" were found in the exact same area. Again it was decided it should be biopsied. On December 9, 1998, I had a stereotactic biopsy at City of Hope. With a machine that looks like a mammogram machine, I stood up, hugged this hunk of steel, and laid my bare breast on the plate, while from above a needle entered my breast and removed a sampling of the tissue. The hospital was using this machine for the first time and the doctor asked me if it was okay if the sales rep, a young guy, stayed while we did the procedure. "Sure, why not." Modesty in this setting seemed pointless.

After the procedure was over Dr. Shaw, the supervising radiologist who read my X-rays, came to the dressing room and said, "I didn't like our aim. We need to do it again." So, a few weeks later, in January 1999, I was back for another stereotactic core biopsy.

The following week Dr. Lawrence Wagman, the oncology surgeon, called me to come in. He wasn't there, however, the day I came in for my results. Instead I met with a young South African doctor. I went to the appointment alone. I remember sitting, numb, on the end of the examining table, the white tissue paper crinkling under my seat. I tried to read his face as he entered the room but his demeanor gave nothing away. He was very tall and emotionless and spoke with a South African accent. We were two strangers about to share a moment I will never forget. I remember his words, the dreaded words. And his expressionless face. "You have cancer. It's malignant." I felt like I was watching a movie of someone else's life.

Now what?

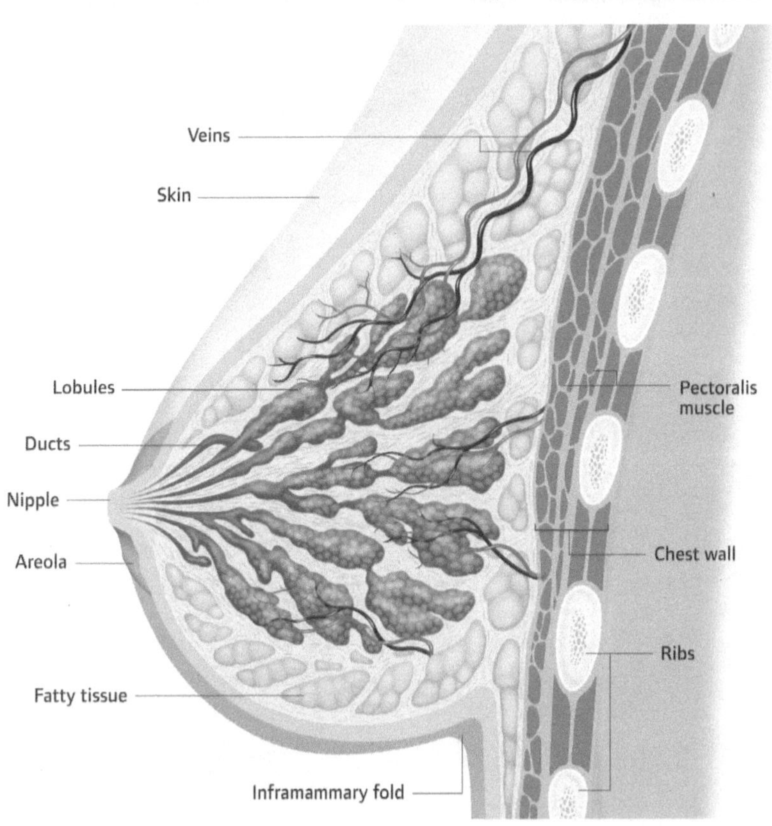

The anatomy of the breast.

2

Now What?

When you are ill, your energy level is quite low, and the intelligence of the organism may take over and use the remaining energy for healing of the body, and so there is not enough left for the mind, that is to say, egoic thinking and emotion.

–Eckhart Tolle, *A New Earth*

In early 1999 what followed were two open biopsies and a sentinel node biopsy at City of Hope in Duarte, California. Once again they didn't get the right spot the first time and so I had two lumpectomies a month apart. The pathological diagnosis was, "ER and PR positive Her2/neu negative with both invasive ductal carcinoma and lobular carcinoma."

The first lumpectomy surgery included a sentinel node biopsy, which tests your sentinel lymph node to try and determine if the cancer has traveled beyond your breast. For that procedure they inject your breast near the biopsy site a couple of hours prior to your surgery with a small dose of radioactive substance and blue dye. That substance travels to the lymph nodes and during surgery they use a Geiger counter (yes a "Geiger counter") to determine the "sentinel node," namely the one or ones the substance travels to first. Those are the ones they remove and test. The advantage of this is that they don't have to take out all your lymph nodes, which is important because lack of lymph nodes can lead to fluid retention in the arm and can become a painful problem (lymphedema). Removing only the pertinent lymph nodes reduces but not necessarily eliminates the risk of this condition occurring.

WHAT IS A BREAST?

The anatomy of the breast is both miraculous and complex. Few parts of the body raise such controversy and have been the object of more attention. What could be more innocent than the place that mother's milk comes from? And yet, due to the way they respond sexually and the way they are responded to sexually, breasts have always held more mystery and been the object of more intense outward attention than many other body parts. "Wardrobe malfunction" is now part of our lexicon because breasts cause such a ruckus. And it is well-documented throughout history that breasts were important. The very galaxy that we live in, The Milky Way, was named by the Greeks because they thought it was Goddess Hera's milk.

And yet, as miraculous as breasts are in their natural state, truckloads of money are spent in order to make them a more idealized version. According to the American Society for Aesthetic Plastic Surgery (ASAPS), there were 318,123 breast augmentations and approximately half as many breast reductions in 2010. Millions upon millions of dollars are spent on cosmetic breast surgery in the U.S. Women as well as men (and maybe because of men) are obsessed, or so it seems, with breasts.

The breast is a combination of nerves, veins, arteries, ducts, glands, lobes, connective tissue, lymph vessels, muscle and

fat. It contains a number of ductal systems, or branches, more like a tree inverted within a breast. Hormones trigger milk production upon giving birth. When a woman breastfeeds, the glands or lobules are the place milk is made and then the ducts transport the milk through the lactiferous sinus to the nipple. A breast is considered "immature" if it has not gone through the event of pregnancy, which changes the architecture of the breast.

Before baby's formula became so commonplace, the human race's existence was dependent upon natural breast milk. Breasts can make blood into life-saving milk. Perhaps part of our strong desire as women to preserve our breasts is linked to this life-giving quality. Even if we have never given birth, or have no plans to do so, we still have the anthropological imprint that our breasts matter. And maybe that accounts for some of the male attention (fixation) on them as well. It wasn't that long ago, historically speaking, that without your mate having healthy breasts (breasts that could produce milk) your offspring would die. Survival of the species is a powerful motivator and it may contribute to the primal male behavioral response to breasts that society likes to sexualize but I believe is underestimated at its core. We have, with baby formula, progressed as a society so that the original design function of breasts, to provide milk for offspring, while still viable and even considered optimal, can be effectively replaced. Still, what has historically always been true for thousands of years is hard to shake and anthropological hard-wiring is formidable.

Breasts have been at the core of our survival as a species. Like all other mammals (so-called because we have mammary glands) we breastfeed our young. What is different in our case is that we have two nipples while other mammals

have multiple nipples known as a milk ridge. We also are different than other mammals in that our breasts develop without relation to our fertility cycle.

In the 1980s I was the production manager for *Vogue* magazine, a place where "female beauty" was constantly being defined and redefined. But I remember clearly that it always included, in every naked image, two healthy symmetrical breasts. We have been strictly taught in modern culture, in addition to our historical predisposition, that breasts, to be beautiful, come in pairs and look and act alike.

Yet when you are defining "what is a breast" in the 21st century you realize the definition in this society is ever-changing. It is no longer just about surviving and breastfeeding, and with augmentation and reconstruction it isn't even about being natural. Where function defined form, form is now often on its own.

WHAT IS THE LYMPHATIC SYSTEM?

The lymphatic system is the highway drainage system that runs throughout the body. This is one of the routes that cancer takes to infiltrate the entire system. Lymph fluid also contains immune system cells that fight infection. In the area of the breasts, lymph vessels are positioned against the chest wall and take lymph (the fluid) to the lymph nodes, which reside under the arm, around the collarbone and in the chest. There are about 30-odd lymph nodes, the size and shape of small beans, located on each side of the breast/chest area. There are more than 500 lymph nodes throughout the entire body.

WHAT IS CANCER?

We talk about cancer as though it has invaded us. But cancer is our abnormal cells gone haywire. They are on a mission to constantly shape-shift and colonize. And in their

unregulated state they act like a bully in the playground, pushing the good cells around. Their abnormal hyper-growth causes cells to form a tumor. Some tumors are benign (non-cancerous) and some tumors are malignant (cancerous). Cancer cells "think" they are immortal. They are an aberration of the normal flow of life and resist the cycle of creation – birth, life and death.

According to the American Cancer Society website, "Normal body cells grow, divide and die in an orderly fashion. During the early years of a person's life, normal cells divide more rapidly until the person becomes an adult. After that, cells in most parts of the body divide only to replace worn-out or dying cells and to repair injuries. Because cancer cells continue to grow and divide, they are different from normal cells. Instead of dying they outlive normal cells and continue to form (more) new abnormal cells."

Through gene analysis, experts can now tell if certain mutations such as the ones found in BRCA 1 or BRCA 2 genes are present that might lead to cancer, but they cannot reliably predict cancer. The alterations found in these genes raises the odds statistically but it does not necessarily lead to a cancer diagnosis although the odds are high. Approximately 87% of women with these gene mutations will get breast cancer in their lifetime.

ARE ALL CANCERS ALIKE?

No. Not even all breast cancers are alike. And the reality is it all depends on how the cancer behaves in the individual patient. Some are fast-growing and more invasive. Others grow slower and stay more contained. Some breast cancers are receptive to hormone therapy while others are not.

The pathology of the cancer will tell you the nature of the breast cancer and tell you the grade of tumor. The higher the grade, the more aggressive the tumor. The complete pathology gives doctors a code by which to talk about and treat it.

WHAT IS IT ABOUT MOST BREAST CANCERS THAT MAKES THEM TREATABLE?

Some breast cancer if caught and excised in its early stages may never recur, depending on the kind of breast cancer you have and how aggressive it is behaving. It can often be detected on a mammogram even when there is no palpable lump. It might show up as "calcifications." On the X-ray they often look like tiny white dots. If there is no palpable lump but it shows up on a mammogram it is likely to be contained in your breast. It's likely, but not always the case, that when caught in the earliest stage it is often highly treatable through surgery, radiation and drug protocol. This is the optimal time at which you want to be diagnosed if possible. The earlier the better as it has a direct impact on your survival. And it is also important to determine at this stage if possible if it has traveled beyond the breast. However, an aggressive tumor could act in an aggressive way no matter when it is detected.

WHAT ARE THE SYMPTOMS OF BREAST CANCER?

Unfortunately, symptoms are often not apparent as breast cancer is most often *painless* and *hidden* in early stages.

However, there are some signs to look out for:

A palpable lump (one you can feel) in the breast or under the arm, above or under the collarbone.

A thickening of part of the breast.

Change in the size or shape of the breast.

Swelling, warmth and/or redness of the breast.

Skin irritation or a dimpling of the skin.

Nipple pain or inversion. Nipple discharge that is not breast milk.

A painful itch in the breast.

These signs don't mean you have breast cancer but they should be discussed with your physician immediately.

Breast cancer is a deadly disease so one would think you would feel ill if you had it. Or that it would be painful. But in the early stages in most instances neither occurs. You generally do not feel bad and you aren't in pain. So why worry? Because it is that which is going on within, left undetected, that can kill you – it is as simple as that. And the odds of having this disease are high – remember *one in eight is the average lifetime risk with some women having even a higher risk.*

Women are used to living with a certain amount of pain and or discomfort. Having a monthly menstrual cycle teaches us that a small amount of pain is not cause for alarm and many of us have learned to tolerate the pain of our period or even the more acute pain of pregnancy. The fact that breast cancer *does not* cause pain in its early stages makes it that much more of a threat. Logical thinking would have you conclude that the absence of pain makes it harmless.

Nothing could be further from the truth.

Breast cancer most often is detected in one breast at a time. Because you have it in one breast doesn't mean you will get it in the other, although with lobular carcinoma the chance of getting it in the other breast is higher.

WHAT IS A CLINICAL BREAST EXAM (CBE)?

A CBE is an exam done by a trained physician or health care professional. Women over the age of 20 should be examined by a professional at least yearly. This is often done during your annual Ob-Gyn appointment. While most breast cancers strike in women over 50, breast cancers in younger women are more aggressive and deadly and therefore the need for monitoring should not be minimized. Also, the physician should take notes and keep a record of any changes and abnormalities. This will help determine if your breasts change from one year to the next and if anything is alarming. Remember that anyone with breast tissue, no matter the age (or gender), is at risk for breast cancer.

WHAT DOES THE TERM "CARCINOMA" MEAN?

"Carcinoma" is another name for cancer.

IS THERE BREAST CANCER (CARCINOMA) THAT IS NON-INVASIVE?

Yes. There are two primary types of breast cancer, non-invasive and invasive. Non-invasive breast cancer is called DCIS or Ductal Carcinoma In-Situ and LCIS or Lobular Carcinoma In-Situ. According to the American Cancer Society there were approximately 67,770 new cases of

non-invasive breast cancer diagnosed in the U.S. in 2008. DCIS and LCIS are both non-invasive cancers. The cancer is contained in the ducts (DCIS) or the lobes (LCIS). However, without treatment both of these can become invasive and infiltrate the surrounding tissue, although DCIS appears to do this more often. DCIS and LCIS are not always apparent on a mammogram, and a breast MRI is better at detecting LCIS.

WHAT IS DUCTAL CARCINOMA IN-SITU (DCIS)?

Ductal Carcinoma In-Situ means the cancer is in the duct but has not broken through the duct wall. It is still "in place" – in-situ. This may still require surgery and radiation treatment.

WHAT IS INFILTRATING DUCTAL CARCINOMA?

This is the most common form of breast cancer found in women: 70% of the cases are Infiltrating Ductal Carcinoma. This means that it started in the ducts and has infiltrated into the surrounding breast tissue. According to the American Cancer Society in 2008 there were an estimated 182,460 new cases of Infiltrating Ductal Carcinoma.

WHAT IS LOBULAR CARCINOMA IN-SITU (LCIS)?

Lobular Carcinoma is a pathological finding that signifies possible increased risk of developing invasive breast cancer. The lobes are tube-like and LCIS would be inside these tubes. When the diagnosis is lobular carcinoma there is often a thickening rather than a lump. "Typically, LCIS has no clinical manifestations and no patho-gnomonic mammographic signs," according to *The M.D. Anderson Cancer Care Series: Breast Cancer*. LCIS also has the reputation

of often being found contra lateral: a finding in one breast often leads to a finding in the other breast.

WHAT IS INFILTRATING LOBULAR CARCINOMA?

This is when the cancer that is in the lobes has broken out and invaded the tissue around the lobes.

WHAT IS INFLAMMATORY BREAST CANCER (IBC)?

In Inflammatory Breast Cancer (IBC) the breast can appear red or swollen or dimpled like the skin of an orange, or the nipple is inverted but this is a rare form and not what most women experience. IBC is, however, an aggressive form and needs to be treated seriously and immediately. Most women have never heard of IBC and due to its aggressive nature it is vital to know the signs.

WHAT ARE SOME OF THE OTHER RARER FORMS OF BREAST CANCER?

Medullary Carcinoma is a rare form of ductal carcinoma.

Paget's disease is a breast cancer of the nipple. In this case the nipple retracts as the tumor grows behind the nipple pulling it inward. This is found in only 1 percent of the women diagnosed with breast cancer.

Phyllodes tumors are a cancer of the connective tissue of the breast. Approximately 25% of these tumors are malignant.

WHAT DOES A BREAST CANCER DIAGNOSIS FROM A BIOPSY MEAN?

A breast cancer diagnosis from a biopsy means you have to make decisions regarding how to excise any cancer that

may be left in the body if you don't have clear margins. If it was a core biopsy then more surgery is necessary. Doctors can't determine if they got it all from a core sample. From this point either the patient will have to undergo a lumpectomy or a mastectomy. This decision is not as clear as one might think. Some women opt for the breast-conserving surgery of a lumpectomy while others, at this juncture, decide that a mastectomy is their best choice. Determining if the cancer has migrated to the lymph nodes is critical and a sentinel node biopsy should be considered. It is possible, if the tumor is large, that they will advise you to have chemotherapy *before* surgery in order to reduce the size of the tumor.

WHAT IS A MAMMOGRAM?

A mammogram is an X-ray of the breast. It can sometimes detect an early breast cancer prior to a lump being felt. While the standard American Cancer Society recommendation is that women 40 and older should have a mammogram every year, if you are younger than that and feel something isn't right or at high-risk, earlier screening might be necessary. Using mammograms for screening purposes has resulted in early detection; however, they are not foolproof. So why am I advocating mammograms when in my case they were unable to detect cancer three different times? Because they are the best we have so far in determining if something is wrong. They are a relatively easy, fast, non-invasive and cost-effective test. That said, they are not always accurate.

The purpose of a mammogram is to detect any abnormality that may need further investigation. This could show up as calcifications which are not palpable or as a lump. One of the issues is that fat and connective tissue appear as white on a mammogram – the same as a tumor. When you have dense

breasts with more connective tissue this can make it harder to locate any tumor or calcifications if they are present.

Women seem to have three basic reasons as to why they haven't gone for a mammogram. First, I've heard said, "I don't want to know if something is wrong." As though not knowing would somehow make it go away. So let me give it to you straight. *Ignorance does not protect you from breast cancer.* The second reason I have heard is that "mammograms hurt." Yes, it is true they aren't comfortable but trust me; breast cancer hurts more, a whole lot more. And third, it costs money. This is an obstacle for many women but there are a few things you can do. You can check around and compare prices. Not all facilities charge the same amount and you can ask them upfront if they will take what your insurance pays as the total amount. You may also be able to negotiate upfront a lower cash fee.

TIP: During a mammogram the breast is compressed while the X-ray is taken. To compress it the technician presses down on an electric pedal – like a sewing machine pedal. If you are nervous about the compression ask the nurse to manually compress you. All mammogram machines have the capability to compress the breast manually and you and the technician will have more control over the compression this way. The denser your breasts, the more they need compression so as to get a more accurate photo of the tissue. There is a reason for the compression but the pain can be minimized if the technician is aware of your sensitivity and does it slowly with manual control.

TIP: During a mammogram you can protect your thyroid by asking the technician for a thyroid shield. Thyroid cancer in women is on the rise and protecting it from

unnecessary X-ray exposure during a dental visit or while getting a mammogram is wise.

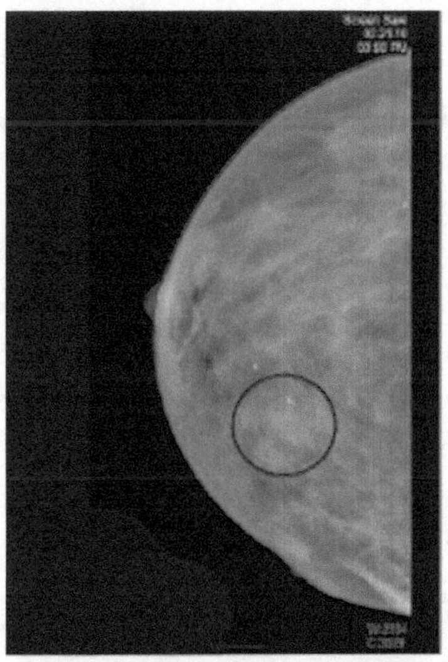

Mammogram X-ray showing malignant calcifications.

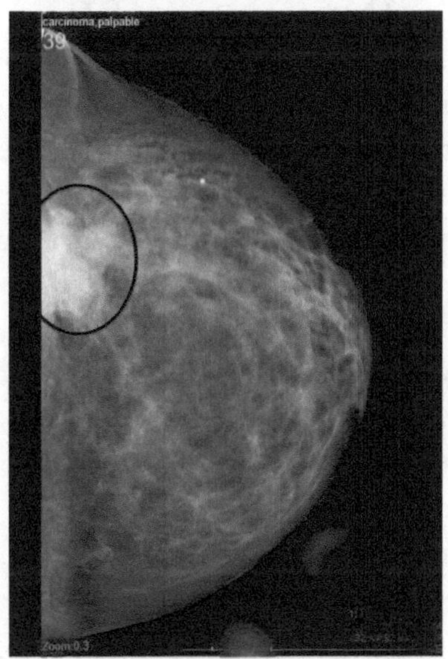

Mammogram X-ray showing a malignant palpable tumor.

WHAT IS DIGITAL MAMMOGRAPHY?

There was a time when if you had a mammogram you had the option of taking the hard films with you. That is still often the case but there is also the newer technology of Digital Mammography where the image is on a computer screen and therefore can be manipulated – enlarged and enhanced – to get a better read and can be delivered through the computer or put on a CD. Digital mammography could be especially helpful if you have dense breasts. Digital mammograms can also be easily transferred as digital files to hospitals and other doctors if necessary. This is an improvement from your having to pick up the X-rays and take them to another doctor. This also makes it easier if you need a second opinion at a different facility. A word of warning: digital mammography has been known to have more false positive results.

WHAT IS MOLECULAR BREAST IMAGING (MBI)?

The future, at least for women with dense breasts and women at higher than normal risk, may be in Molecular Breast Imaging, which is FDA approved as of 2010 but it is not as widely available as mammograms. This test involves gamma rays (not X-rays) and an injection of a short-lived radioactive tracer that would light up a tumor. MBI is being developed at the Mayo Clinic in Rochester, Minnesota. It did originally administer about 10 times the radiation as a mammogram, but the developers have worked to reduce this amount and now the radiation dose is similar to that of a digital mammogram.

One aspect that is highly positive about this test is that it is far easier to read than a regular mammogram. According to Dr. Deborah Rhodes, the Director of Mayo Clinic's Executive Health Program, as she explained during a TED conference in 2010, "MBI exploits the different molecular behaviors of tumors." She emphasizes that women need to know their "breast density" as it has an impact on how readable and accurate their individual mammograms may be and also on their risk status. Higher density equals greater risk.

WHAT IS AN ULTRASOUND?

An ultrasound is a non-invasive procedure that yields an internal picture of your breast. It uses high-frequency sound waves to determine if a lump is solid or liquid. A cold gel is put on your breast and then a smooth paddle is rubbed over the gel. Sound waves are sent through the breast. If the waves encounter something solid (a tumor or a benign mass) the waves bounce back. If they encounter something liquid, like a cyst, the waves penetrate. It is a completely non-invasive, painless test and a good step in determining the nature of any abnormality. Usually it is requested after a mammogram if there is something suspicious on the films. In the case of a younger patient the breasts are sometimes so dense they are hard to read on a mammogram. Even if there is a solid mass it does not mean that it is cancer. Another test may be needed to determine the nature of the mass.

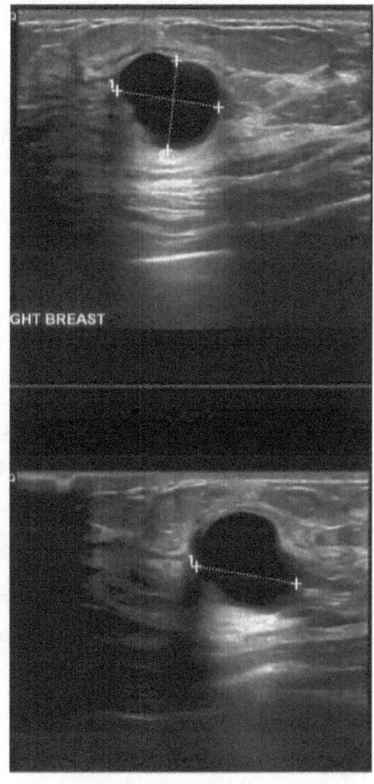

Ultrasound showing a malignant tumor.

WHAT IS A BREAST MRI WITH OR WITHOUT CONTRAST?

MRI or Magnetic Resonance Imaging uses a large magnet and radio waves to get an exact picture of the breast. It measures the blood supply. During an MRI a technician may give you an IV so that they can administer dye (contrast). This will allow them to get a more detailed image of the vessels. MRI is sometimes used prior to surgery or can be helpful in women with dense breasts. And can it be used after breast cancer to determine if there is any recurrence.

A breast MRI does lead to more false positive results. It is also used to determine the extent of the disease and see if there is any infiltration into the chest wall. And it is sometimes used to document the effectiveness of chemotherapy. Whenever physicians plan to use IV contrast or dye, they will likely check blood tests to assess your kidney function, since contrast can have a negative effect on your kidneys.

WHAT IS AN FNA?

An FNA is a fine needle aspiration. If there is a lump or area that has been determined to be questionable then the doctor might perform an FNA. A regular-size needle would be inserted in the area and a small amount of material would be drawn out and then put on slides to be examined under a microscope. It is a relatively simple procedure and although not foolproof a good step in determining if something abnormal is going on. Again, if after this test you still feel something isn't right, discuss it with your doctor.

WHAT IS A CORE BIOPSY?

A core biopsy takes out a small sample of the tissue of the breast. Usually this is done while the doctor is guided by ultrasound. The area is anesthetized with lidocaine or similar numbing agent and then a gun-like mechanism shoots a hollow cylinder into your breast and a sample of tissue retracts into the gun. The tissue sample is then sent to a lab for diagnosis. Core biopsies are frequently done if calcifications are found on a mammogram; in that case, an X-ray of the biopsied material will confirm if all the calcifications were removed. It is an invasive procedure and many things need to be considered prior to having a core biopsy. If it is breast cancer, a core biopsy should confirm that but there is the chance that the doctor will miss testing the actual tumor site. This also blasts the area and disturbs what is growing there – not the best of circumstances if in fact it is cancer. So while a core biopsy can give you a positive diagnosis it isn't always accurate if it is negative. And, in the event that the doctor did miss the tumor, the area is now traumatized and still growing and the scar tissue makes it that much more difficult to tell if it is cancer in the future. It is a diagnostic procedure, not a treatment.

WHAT IS A LUMPECTOMY?

A lumpectomy or open biopsy is the removal of the section of your breast with the tumor in order to get clear margins (the area around the tumor). The size of the lumpectomy will depend on the size of the tumor. This is done in a hospital, usually under sedation. Depending on the time of day your surgery takes place and whether a sentinel node biopsy is planned you may or may not spend the night in the hospital.

WHAT IS A CT OR CAT SCAN?

A CT or CAT scan is a Computerized Tomography scan. This is necessary when a more detailed view is needed or to determine if there has been any spread of the disease to the bone, liver, lung or lymph nodes.

WHAT IS A PET SCAN?

A PET scan is a Positron Emission Tomography scan. Prior to the test you will be given a radioactive IV with glucose and you might also take oral contrast at the same time to enhance the gastrointestinal system. This scan distinguishes the body's reaction to sugar in the body. Normally the body absorbs sugar and turns it into energy. Cancer cells absorb more sugar than normal cells. On the computer screen, hot spots will be present if there are areas where more sugar than usual is being absorbed by the cells. The more sugar and larger the hot spot, the more likely it is cancer. This test helps determine if the cancer has spread to other organs.

TIP: Now, at the latest, is the time to start your Health Notebook. That way if something abnormal shows up in the future, you will have a notebook from now on containing your reports, doctor visits and documents of other health issues. Looking back, I'd say age 40 is a good time to start one of these books even if all is well. Time passes so quickly and you forget what happened and where. Having it documented makes everything easier.

TIP: If you are having a breast MRI with contrast, the injection of the dye and radioactive material can be painful. Ask for a numbing agent such as lidocaine beforehand. If your request is met with a protest as mine was, with the nurse saying, "Well then I will have to stick you twice," insist on it anyway. At the very least ask for numbing cream.

TIP: If you are scheduled for a lumpectomy, ask the surgeon about a Sentinel Node Biopsy and if it will be performed in addition to the lumpectomy.

WHAT IS A SENTINEL NODE BIOPSY?

Checking the lymph nodes is the way to determine if the cancer has spread beyond the breast. Your lymph system is the body's drainage system. You have a virtual highway of drainage in your body and your lymph nodes are the toll booths. You have about 30 odd lymph nodes around one side of your collarbone and under your arm. A Sentinel Node Biopsy removes the first few of these in the path to be tested, hence the word "sentinel." Fluid is drained via your lymph system and nodes are the inceptors of cells that would contain the cancer.

If cancer has not made it to your lymph system it is considered contained in the breast. If it is found in your lymph system the cancer is no longer contained and is considered systemic. If it shows up in your lymph system you will almost always undergo chemotherapy. Not news you want to hear, I know, but this is information that you must know. You absolutely must get a handle on where it has traveled thus far in order for the treatment to have an opportunity to be efficient and effective. And then there are the situations where it does not show up in your lymph nodes but is found in a distant site elsewhere in the body. This is rare but it does happen, so a sentinel node biopsy is not 100% reliable. In the past surgeons would have removed all the nodes but they have been able to reduce the number to the most pertinent through this procedure.

With a few lymph nodes being removed there is a chance of lymphedema but that is less likely with only a few nodes being removed and the information they yield is essential. As a result of this procedure you may find yourself temporarily with a large egg-like sack of fluid under your arm, referred to as a seroma after surgery. It can be

alarming and painful but it can be easily drained by your doctor. It may take more than one time for your doctor to drain the deposit of fluid and your body to adjust and absorb the remaining fluid.

WHAT IS AN AXILLARY NODE DISSECTION?

If cancer is found in the lymph nodes or is suspected to be there, an Axillary Node Dissection will likely be done. In this procedure the surgeon would remove almost all the lymph nodes under the arm on the side of the cancer. Generally the nodes would then be tested to see how many nodes are positive for cancer, if any. This information would be important in determining the stage of the cancer.

For my first surgery in January 1999 I was advised to spend the night since I would be undergoing both a sentinel node biopsy and a lumpectomy. I drove myself to City of Hope and arrived at 5:30 A.M. It was chilly and still dark outside. I had never had surgery at a hospital before for anything serious, other than an emergency operation due to a bad skiing accident in France in my twenties (on my honeymoon by the way). In that situation I was made unconscious on the mountain and airlifted by helicopter so, while very dramatic, I had never experienced the "anxiety of waiting" before.

In the early morning the hospital had an eerily quiet quality to it with very few people around, just the buzz of fluorescent lights humming in the background. A 12-year-old girl with an amputated leg sat in a wheelchair with her mom in the reception area. She was suffering from bone cancer and about to have her fourth or fifth surgery. She seemed old beyond her years. Her skin was pasty white and she wore a blue cap which covered her head. She resonated maturity to such a degree it made the teddy bear she was holding appear incongruous. She talked with her mom about what she was going to do after the surgery. She wanted to go to the amusement park Magic Mountain. A promise was made. I still think about her.

I recall being taken back to the pre-op area and struggling to hold it together. A nice nurse looked in on me and then returned with tissues. Dr. Wagman came in with his head covered in what looked like an oversized shower cap and glasses. He was reassuring and asked me if I had any questions. I didn't because I really didn't know what to ask or expect. I woke up in the recovery room shivering and shaking. I have since learned to ask for plenty of warm blankets.

TIP: Before the surgery ask for warm blankets to be provided for you post-op in the recovery room. Your body temperature drops so low that you feel like you will never be warm again. Hospitals are now much more aware of the risks of hypothermia (low body temperature) that can accompany procedures and have gotten better about treating and preventing it, but you may still have to ask.

After the surgery I shared a room with a woman who was dying of ovarian cancer. It was quiet and dark on my side. I was closer to the hall door. The curtain between us was pulled but the lights on my side were off since I had told no one I was there, so no one would be visiting, plus I was too groggy to read – no reason for lights. I could see shadows through the curtain, as if a play were being performed just a few feet away.

I only saw her face a couple of times when I got up to use the bathroom. I didn't want to look in her direction as her husband was there with her keeping vigil, sitting in a straight-back wooden chair. I felt like I was in their bedroom. I shouldn't be there for these private matters. He hardly moved and said little. He reminded me of one of those life-size stuffed people, although somewhat deflated, as his shoulders slumped. I remember her muffled voice and occasional tears coming from her as nurses and hospice personnel attended to her and made arrangements to move her to a hospice care facility. The light above her bed illuminated the white turban she had on her head covering her baldness and her pale white translucent face under it. Around 10:00 P.M. I was given a sleeping pill. Sometime in the night they moved her as she was gone in the morning. I wondered how much more time she had.

Note: Why can't hospitals see that offering private rooms for those on the verge of hospice is the right thing to do?

In the morning when I was ready to leave, I called and got a wheelchair sent to the room. I wheeled myself to the pharmacy, picked up my pain medicine, and wheeled myself outside. Against hospital policy, I drove myself home.

TIP: Never leave the hospital alone. While you may feel fine at first you can have a latent reaction to the surgery.

TIP: When preparing for surgery give some thought to having "light" food available when you come home. It is likely you won't feel like eating much but you may be on pain medicine and therefore need something in your stomach to buffer the drugs.

The diagnosis was cancer – "invasive ductal carcinoma and lobular ductal carcinoma" – and the margins were not clear enough which meant I had to have another lumpectomy a month later. The bad news was that I had cancer in both the ducts and the lobules. The good news was that it was node negative (my lymph nodes were clear). The official diagnosis was "ER and PR positive, Her2/neu negative with both invasive ductal carcinoma and lobular carcinoma and node negative." Another lumpectomy and radiation were recommended due to the early stage of the tumor and the fact I was node negative.

For the next surgery I was in and out the same day as it was just on the breast and not the lymph nodes. Due to the malignancy, I had to follow these surgeries with seven weeks of radiation. My pathology staging was (T1aN0).

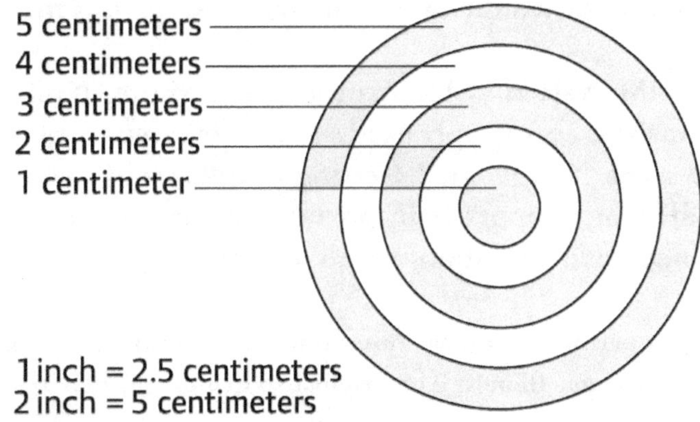

Sizes of a tumor measured in centimeters.

STAGING OF BREAST CANCER

Staging is a way of describing the advancement of the cancer based on the pathology of the cancer. It indicates where, how large, and what kind of cancer it is, and if it is affecting other organs or parts of the body. Staging is used in deciding treatment and also prognosis. The pathology report would indicate the nature of the cancer and from this the doctor would determine which stage it is in.

The TNM system (which measures Tumors, Nodes and Metastasis) is commonly used so doctors can communicate in the same "language." Getting familiar with what is on the pathology report is important so that you can make informed decisions about your treatment.

Used with permission of the American Joint Committee on Cancer (AJCC), Chicago, Illinois. The original source of this material is the AJCC Cancer Staging Manual Seventh Edition (2010) published by Springer Science and Business Media LLC, www.springer.com

THE PATHOLOGY REPORT

T for tumor, N for node involvement and M for metastasis. Stage zero (0) and stages I through IV (stages 1 through 4).

TX – At this time the tumor cannot be evaluated. This could be the case when calcifications are seen on a mammogram but no mass.

T0 – There is no obvious cancer evident in the breast.

TIS – IS refers to "in situ" which means it is confined to the breast area that is identified.

DCIS – This can refer to what is known as DCIS (Ductal Carcinoma In-Situ) which is considered a precursor to

breast cancer. This would be found in the ducts but has not spread beyond to other tissue. It can later develop into an invasive breast cancer (Invasive Ductal Carcinoma).

LCIS – This is Lobular Carcinoma In Situ. This refers to abnormal cells being found in the lobules and glands.

T1 – The tumor in the breast is 2 centimeters or smaller.

T1mic – The tumor in the breast is 2 centimeters or smaller and some cancer cells have been found in the surrounding tissue but they are not larger than 1 centimeter. Mic refers to micro invasion – or some invasion to the surrounding tissue.

T1a – The tumor is larger than .1 centimeter but smaller than .5 centimeters.

T1b – The tumor is larger than .5 centimeters but smaller than 1 centimeter.

T1c – The tumor is larger than 1 centimeter but not larger than 2 centimeters.

T2a – The tumor is less than 2 cm and/or lymph nodes under the arm are involved.

T2b – The tumor is larger than 2 cm, but less than 5cm and the lymph nodes under the arm are involved OR the tumor is larger than 5 cm but the underarm lymph nodes are not involved.

T3 – The tumor is larger than 5 centimeters.

T4 – The tumor has spread to the chest wall or to the skin. This is also the diagnosis for Inflammatory Breast Cancer, a rare but serious type of breast cancer.

T4a – The cancer has spread to the chest wall.

T4b – Indicates there are external and more obvious symptoms showing on the skin. There could be swelling in the area or what is known as "peau d'orange" where the skin is pitted like the skin of an orange. Often the area would be painful.

T4c – Both T4a and T4b would be present.

T4d – This indicates an inflammatory form of breast cancer where the breast is warm, distorted or red. This is an aggressive form of cancer. Aside from the tumor there is lymph node involvement, which needs to be determined. This "involvement" would indicate where the cancer has spread.
N stands for Node. Lymph nodes are a filtration system for the body. Lymph nodes go on alert and swell when infection is present. There are many lymph nodes located under the arm and top of the chest area, around the collarbone and breast bone. In breast cancer these would be the "regional" lymph nodes. Other lymph nodes in the body would be considered "distant" sites in terms of the breast cancer. The ones under the arm are the "axillary nodes."

NX – The lymph nodes cannot be or have not been evaluated.

N0 – The lymph nodes have been tested and there is no lymph node involvement.

N1 – The cancer has spread to one to three of the lymph nodes under the arm.

N2 – The cancer has spread to four to nine of the lymph nodes under the arm or elsewhere in the regional area.

N2a – The cancer has spread to four to nine of the lymph nodes under the arm and the size of at least one of the tumors is 2 millimeters.

N2b – The cancer has spread to the regional mammary lymph nodes but is not found under the arm.

N3 – The cancer has spread to more than 10 lymph nodes.

N3a – The cancer has spread to more than 10 lymph nodes under the arm or to the infraclavicular (under the collarbone) lymph nodes.

N3b – The cancer has spread to 10 or more lymph nodes and includes the mammary nodes and the axillary nodes (under the arm).

N3c – The cancer has spread to the supraclavicular lymph nodes.

M refers to "metastasis." Metastasis means the cancer has traveled beyond the breast to other parts of the body. Metastatic breast cancer is still breast cancer even if it is found in the bone, liver or brain.

MX – There has been a spread that cannot be or has not been determined.

M0 – The disease has not metastasized.

M1 – It has been determined that the cancer has metastasized to another part of the body beyond the breast. It is still breast cancer even though it has traveled elsewhere in the body from its origins in the breast.

The pathology will then be combined and the staging will be determined.

STAGE 0

Ductal carcinoma in situ or non-invasive breast cancer.

STAGE I

The tumor is small (less than 2 centimeters) and has not spread to the lymph nodes.

STAGE IIa

The tumor is smaller than or equal to 2 centimeters and has spread to the lymph nodes under the arm (T1, T1mic, N1, and M0).

The tumor is larger than 2 centimeters but not larger than 5 centimeters and has not spread to the lymph nodes (T2, N0, M0).

There is no evidence of cancer in the breast but there is cancer in the lymph nodes (T0, N1, M0).

STAGE IIb

The tumor is larger than 2 centimeters but not larger than 5 centimeters and has spread to the lymph nodes under the arm (T2, N1, M0).

The tumor is larger than 5 centimeters but has not spread to the lymph nodes under the arm (T3, N0, M0).

STAGE IIIa

The tumor is smaller than 5 centimeters and has spread to the axillary lymph nodes (under the arm) (T1, N2, M0 or T2, N2, M0).

The tumor is larger than 5 centimeters and has spread to the lymph nodes (T3, N1, M0 or T3, N2, M0).

STAGE IIIb

The tumor has spread to the chest wall, caused swelling or ulceration or may be diagnosed as IBC – Inflammatory Breast Cancer. It has not spread to other parts of the body.

STAGE IIIc

A tumor of any size has not spread to distant parts of the body but has spread to the lymph nodes in the N3 group.

Stage IV

The tumor can be any size and has spread to distant sites in the body. The common sites for spread are the bone, brain, liver, lungs or chest wall (any T, any N, M1).

Once the staging is determined a treatment plan will be prescribed.

WHAT IS A MEDICAL ONCOLOGIST AND WHAT ARE TUMOR MARKERS?

A medical oncologist is a doctor specializing in the chemistry of cancer. He or she will evaluate the tumor markers and determine the chemotherapy or hormonal blocking treatment that may be needed. If your tumor is hormone positive (not all cancers are), it means it will likely be sensitive to hormone treatment such as tamoxifen or aromatase inhibitors.

The tissue from the biopsy will also be evaluated for tumor markers. Tumor markers are proteins on the outside of the tumor and indicate how the tumor will be treated. They also reveal if the cancer is hormone receptive (HR). Most breast cancers are estrogen (ER+) and progesterone (PR+) positive – meaning they need these hormones to grow. Some breast cancers are HR negative. HR positive cancers are known to grow slower than HR negative cancers. According to the book, *The M.D. Anderson Cancer Care Series: Breast Cancer*, "Another protein, pS2, is identified within the subset of ER-positive tumors with a particularly favorable outlook."

WHAT IS HER-2/neu?

HER-2/neu is a breast cancer protein. You can be HER-2/neu negative or HER-2/neu positive. HER-2/neu negative cancers are generally known to respond to chemotherapy better than HER-2/neu positive. "Amplification or over expression of HER-2/neu has been associated with poor prognosis in patients with breast cancer and both positive and negative lymph nodes," as stated in *The M.D. Anderson Cancer Care Series: Breast Cancer*.

WHAT IS TRIPLE NEGATIVE?

While most breast cancers (70%) are hormone sensitive (positive), some are not hormone sensitive (negative). If you are progesterone negative (PR-), estrogen negative (ER-) and HER-2/neu negative (Her/2neu-) you may hear it referred to as "triple negative." Your course of treatment will likely differ from breast cancers that are hormone sensitive. Surgery, radiation and chemotherapy are the

treatment modalities currently available for triple negative patients. About 15% of the breast cancer cases in America carry a triple negative diagnosis.

WHAT IS RADIATION?

Radiation is the use of X-rays to kill cancer cells. Sometimes it is used after surgery to kill the microscopic remains and sometimes it is used prior to surgery to shrink the tumor. It is sometimes also used when the cancer has spread to a distant site, such as the spine, in order to shrink the tumor and alleviate pain in the new location. External radiation (EBRT) is the most common treatment for breast cancer patients. Generally you will receive between 180 and 200 rads (CentiGrays) per day. A total dose over the span of treatment depends on your diagnosis but it can be anywhere between 3400 and 7000 rads, depending on if you receive an extra dose to the area where the tumor was located. This is usually administered over a period of weeks.

High Dose Radiation Therapy (HDRT) Brachytherapy is internal radiation, requiring the placement of a capsule or wire inside you to emit radiation in a localized area. A 5-day dose is a typical protocol.

Some centers in Europe now also offer intra-operative radiation therapy, performed at the same time as the procedure to remove the tumor.

Every weekday, for seven weeks, I drove myself to City of Hope, about 50 minutes each way from my home, for treatment. When you are getting radiation you are undressed (at least from the waist up) and it is usually chilly. Due to the type of equipment and the necessary shielding, radiation departments are often in the basement floors, and they always seem to up the air conditioning to keep the machines cool, and so it is at City of Hope too.

For someone who does not have much experience in a medical environment, just seeing these machines alone can be enough to raise your anxiety level. This fact is generally lost on the medical caretaking community, who is accustomed to buzzing machines, strong smells, and patients with needles in their arms and drains coming out of their bodies and masked personnel in official white lab coats.

On the first day of radiation, the technicians measured me and wanted to tattoo me with permanent dots. I didn't want tattoos. They said, "You have to have them." I asked why they couldn't put marks on me that are semi-permanent. Reluctantly they responded, "Well, yes that is an option." Finally they agreed to put bullet size band-aids on me that had to stay on the whole time I was being radiated. I had to replace them carefully after bathing in the exact same place. It was better than tattoos but they only did it because I insisted. My state of mind was when this was over I wanted as few reminders as possible. Sounds a bit silly now, considering what has happened since, but I think it was part of my defiance. I may have breast cancer but you're not going to mark me one second before it is absolutely necessary!

I was told to get undressed and was given a tight, cropped, white fishnet top to put on in order to keep my breasts in the proper, upright position. It was sleeveless, with a bare midriff. I was a hundred and twenty-five pounds, 5'7" with large natural breasts; all I needed was a pole and I could have made some serious cash. I put the tight cropped top on and covered myself with a hospital gown. The technician was a young guy in his twenties and the first day it was a little embarrassing as I unrobed. The room looked like something out of a sci-fi movie, with its clean white shiny floor, cold temperature and a fiberglass bed – very *Avatar*-like. The radiation machine they used on me was enormous. After measuring me and lining up my body, the technician and the nurse would leave me, the door would click shut and alone in the room I would get zapped. All I heard was the sound of the machine – a dull buzzing. For about 15 minutes rads of radiation would enter my body to kill the errant cancer cells. I had to lie perfectly still. It isn't at all painful, just psychologically stressful. My mind raced, "Are they aiming right? Hope they aren't hurting my heart." This went on every weekday for seven weeks.

TIP: During radiation you will be alone in the room but you will be able to communicate with the staff by microphone. And while it is eerie, the actual radiation doesn't hurt. It does come with side effects and everyone responds differently. The skin can appear as though it has been sunburned. Fatigue is also something most women experience. It is hard to know if this lethargy is from the actual radiation or the emotional toll of having cancer and going for daily treatments while juggling the rest of life.

Luckily my skin didn't burn from the radiation. However, some women really suffer with a burning of the skin. This seems especially true with older patients. Over time (years later) that breast did get slightly smaller, which always reminded me of the trauma it went through. I always thought of it as the "brave one." Clearly radiation wasn't "harmless."

During the treatment I was worried the radiation would permanently damage my heart as the cancer was located right over my heart. I was afraid of the cancer but not so afraid that I wasn't conscious of the side effects of treatment. When the doctors told me I had the option of having a boost (additional radiation) in that particular area I declined due to added risk to my heart.

WHAT IS A RADIATION BOOST?

A boost of radiation is an extra dose (approximately between 1000 and 2000 rads) targeted to the site where the tumor is located.

Weeks passed. I recall walking into City of Hope Hospital on one particular day for my radiation treatment. The fountain outside was operating and there were a few patients, all in wheelchairs, getting some air or waiting to be picked up. I remember thinking, "Will I die here? I don't want to die here. I want to be doing something fun when I die – not in a hospital bed."

3

Second Opinion

On the simplest level nothing comes between patient and doctor like a mistake.

– Atul Gawande M.D., *Complications*

In March of 1999, post-radiation, I went alone for a second opinion regarding further treatment options at UCLA Medical Center. It was in a clinic-like setting, with about 10 patients sitting around a long conference table with his or her spouse or companion. I felt the eyes of everyone in the room darting about. Who are the patients, who are the companions, who are the doctors? It was one of the most uncomfortable rooms I have ever been in. I felt exposed and still don't understand the reason for doing this in a group setting as it seemed to fly in the face of privacy issues. After the group session offering general information, I was put in a private room and doctors from the various specialties examined me and reviewed my case. The second opinion from UCLA just confirmed City of Hope's treatment plan.

TIP: Getting a second opinion is just that...a *second* opinion. It should be considered on its merits with no special intrinsic value just because it is second. Sometimes we seek out a second opinion because we don't want to believe the first one and are looking for a different one.

Sometimes we are looking for confirmation. In any case, you are completely within your rights to seek out another opinion, and ethical professionals understand your desire to do so. Any pressure by doctors that this is somehow a waste of your time is unethical. You have every right to gather more information.

You naturally wonder when you get the diagnosis, "How long have I had the cancer?" If you have a lump, the estimates are that it has been growing for six to ten years according to the NBCC (National Breast Cancer Coalition), but of course there is no way of actually knowing exactly when it began.

Although I had a scar from the lumpectomies, at this point my breast was not deformed or changed significantly. However this experience did make me think a lot about how I really felt about my breasts. Sexuality, sensuality, and the reason for attention from guys and women alike – they were a source of envy and interest. How much of my identity as a woman is in my D-cup, Scarlett Johansson-like breasts? I live in Los Angeles where D-cups can be bought for a few thousand dollars, but the real ones are rarer and I knew it. It gave me a certain power and it propelled my self-esteem. How would it be to have them vanish? Scarred? Not real? Not warm? Nipple-less? Not beautiful?

In my twenties I read Betty Rollin's book *First You Cry*, a heart-felt accounting about her experience with breast cancer and coping with the disease. She was a very well-known broadcaster during a time when female role models were rare, so any story by a working woman in the media about a woman's issue intrigued me. I distinctly remember a few salient features of her book: her denial, her panic, her courage and her humor; and now, going through this myself, I know that all four are components of coping. I had also read Gilda Radner's book, *It's Always Something*, and even though it wasn't about breast cancer it hit similar chords – anger, sadness, courage, humor and the need for love. Why I read these books when cancer wasn't on my radar screen I'm not certain. Perhaps an "inner knowing" that something like this may be ahead of me? Or, more likely, just my desire to seek out stories of women coping with and overcoming adversity. If they can manage cancer with grace and humor, I can deal with a difficult boyfriend or a job. I wanted to learn from their example of strength and grace. My singular quest at the time was how do you become a strong woman and make your own way in the world? In the 1970s that was not readily apparent. And, I admired their sense of humor. Humor should not be underestimated as studies have shown laughter heals. Norman Cousins in his famous book, *An Anatomy of an Illness,* talks about how laughter helped relieve his pain.

Which reminds me of a joke my friend Pam tells about a shoe salesman with a foot fetish. The department store was upset that he was fondling women's feet so they transferred him to the sweater department. A few weeks later a woman tried on a sweater and when she came out of the dressing room he drew huge circles on top of her breasts. She looked at him horrified and then looked at the circles and said, "Why did you do that?" He explained to her, "They are for the pockets." Outraged she said, "But I don't want pockets on my sweater." He went over to her, put his hands on her breasts and said, "Okay." He rubbed the lines off her sweater and obviously was rubbing her breasts, "No pockets." That became a tag line whenever we were making breast jokes: "Noooooo pockets."

The previous January, in 1998, my mother was diagnosed with small cell (oat cell) lung cancer. In August of 1998 I went back to New Jersey to care for her along with my brother, Tom. We took her to our brother Fred's house in Michigan so that she could have chemotherapy under his supervision at the hospital he was affiliated with. There was a moment just before her diagnosis when I thought about telling everyone what had been going on with me, but after she was diagnosed I didn't want her to worry about me too, so I decided to just keep it to myself. Besides I was fine or so I thought.

The following year, in August of '99, I went back to New Jersey again to take care of my mom as she now needed constant care. I was there for three weeks and realized I needed to be there full-time. I flew back to California and placed a small ad in *Variety* to rent out my house temporarily. Almost instantly David Boreanaz, the handsome actor, answered the ad. At the time he was starring in the show "Angel" and going through a divorce and needed a temporary place to stay. When he showed up on my doorstep it did make me think, "Holy cow, I should do this more often." David rented my house and so with "Angel" in my house I returned to New Jersey.

I arrived back at Newark airport in August 1999 with my dog, Cinder, not knowing how long I would need to stay. As I waited in the airport for the dog crate to come off the plane, a woman came up to me and said, "Are you Susan Armenti?" I thought, "Gee, I've only been in New Jersey five minutes and already someone knows me." I grew up in central New Jersey where my family has owned a very popular deli business for over 50 years and my uncle was a well-known politician, so people knowing your name and family was not unusual. This however was surprising. Then she said, "I'm Mary, from the deli, Tom sent us." With that she and her husband helped me with my luggage and the dog and we all piled into the pick-up truck and went back to Hamilton, New Jersey. My brother, busy at the deli, had asked them to pick me up but I didn't get the message he wasn't coming. This trip was going to be full of the unexpected and that was just the beginning. I stayed at my mom's house, and it was eerie to be there without her, a precursor of things to come.

That evening I went to see my mom at the nursing home. I didn't want to leave Cinder, my 2-year-old black-and-white cocker spaniel, alone at the house after her traumatic day of travel so I brought her to the Princeton complex. I walked in with

Cinder on her red leash. I guess my maternal demeanor indicated to everyone she was "my child" or might as well be. No one stopped me. As I walked into my mom's room my heart stopped. She looked much thinner than the last time that I had seen her only a week ago. The cancer was taking its toll.

I think the first thing she said to me was, "You had to bring her?" referring to my dog. She wasn't a dog lover and thought it rather horrific that I had brought Cinder into the nursing home. My mom then asked me for water but the water in the sink was turned off due to flooding in the building. I had to go to the nurses' station to get it. I thought, "Great...what am I going to do with Cinder?" I was trying to be inconspicuous and not get thrown out of the place on my first day. I tied Cinder to my mother's bedpost at the foot of the bed and went to the nurses' station to get the water. As I came back into the room Cinder was on her way to pulling my mother's bed (which was on rollers) into the hallway to look for me. It is an image I will never forget. One of those scenes you couldn't have made up. When I left the nursing home that night a frail woman sitting in a wheelchair out in the hall looked up from her dazed state and, seeing Cinder, gave me a huge, dog-loving toothless smile. Cinder "smiled" back. A good reminder one person's agitation is another person's medicine.

For those of you who are in or have ever been in this kind of intensive care-taking situation you know how draining it can be. Every day, just making your way to the hospital becomes the focus. Dealing with doctors, nurses, which tests, what drugs, and then trying to make someone who is ill, or even more emotionally challenging, someone who is dying, more comfortable, all of it is exhausting. When it goes on for weeks or months or years a certain kind of numbness can overcome you. When I have been in these situations it has forced me to be present. The uncertainty of the days underlines the truth, that it is the thinnest of threads that keeps us tethered to this physical world, a world we so often take for granted.

In the nursing home my mom shared a room with someone I will call Bella out of respect for her privacy. She was a rather large sweet elderly woman who, as it turned out, had owned a local sewing store. My mom and I used to frequent the place often taking me there after school to get fabric and thread. Bella lived alone, had no family nearby and had been brought in by ambulance Sunday night. She didn't have any of her belongings with her, not even a change of clothes. I knew my mom still had some of my dad's clothes at home that might fit her, so during the week I brought her one of my dad's pink golf shirts, which she put on immediately, and some toiletries she had requested. I remember she was grateful and knowing how sick my mom was, she was very respectful of our time together in the shared space. And I no doubt found some comfort in seeing that pink golf shirt across the room.

This Princeton nursing home had a good reputation and, as these places go, is very "nice." One day a friend of my mother's came by, Val, to visit and commented to her, "Pat, this place is like the Ritz." My mother, in true tell-it-like-it-is fashion, didn't miss a beat, and told her what she really thought. "Shit Ritz!"

My mom struggled with her small cell lung cancer for the textbook amount of time – 18 months. The Wednesday before she died was a beautiful fall day in New Jersey and she hadn't been outside in weeks. I put her in a wheelchair, covered her in blankets and took her outside the nursing home for some fresh air. She was less than 100 pounds. She noticed and commented on all the colors: the white bench, the yellow tree and the blue sky. She said my name that day. It was the last day my mom spoke.

On Saturday her friends, the "Club girls," women she has known since high school, visited the nursing home. I knew my brother Tom and his wife Noreen would be visiting that night so early evening I went to her church, St. Gregory's the Great, to see if I could find the priest whom she was so fond of, Father Rich. It was near 5 o'clock mass so I thought someone would be around the church at that hour on a Saturday. As I walked into the vestibule there was a priest standing there. I asked him, "Do you know where I could find Father Rich?"As if he were waiting for me, he said, "I'm Father Rich." I introduced myself and he immediately asked about my mom. I asked if he could come see her as I knew his visit would mean a lot to her. He told me he couldn't come that night but would as soon as he could. I thanked him and left.

The next morning around 11:00 A.M. I was in my mom's room at the nursing home and was rereading all the cards she had received, and who walked in but Father Rich. It was Sunday morning and he has a huge congregation, so I said surprised, "It's Sunday, I didn't expect to see you." He looked over at my mom in the bed and said, "I did the early shift so I could come see Pat." He gave me a very gentle smile and walked to her bedside. She wasn't talking at this point but when she saw Father Rich she nearly levitated off the bed, she was so happy to see him. They prayed together.

That night my friend Pam came down from Montclair and stayed in the hospital with me as we kept my mom company. We had a somber dinner together, both of us knowing it wasn't going to be long now.

My mom died the next morning on October 4, 1999. And yes, there were many moments when I wanted to tell her what was going on with me, but I knew it would have made her worry and sad, so I didn't. They had moved Bella out of the room the night before but the crumpled pink golf shirt was left on the bed.

TIP: The days are long when you are taking care of someone who is dying but in my opinion it is also one of the privileges of life, to be present during the transition. My experience, in retrospect, is that if you can slow down enough, those days are precious. As my friend Kim Hahn would say, "Be there, if you can, for the hello and the goodbye."

Sensing perhaps that I was moving on and wanting to be supportive, my former boyfriend, Michael, came to visit me in New Jersey that November. There remained a strong connection between us and while we still loved each other he had missed so much of my life. His visit moved the relationship back into limbo and my sense was that I should and would ultimately return to California – but not yet.

In December, while I was clearing out my mom's house and getting my spirit restored, daughters of my mother's friends asked if I wanted to go out with them one night. It had been months since I had had a girl's night out so I said sure. It was my dad's birthday, December 11. As luck would have it, I met a young beautiful guy that night, I will call him Rob, and ended up having a sweet romance. He was 15 years younger than I was and so handsome. I vacillated about staying in New Jersey and continuing my life there but on New Year's Day 2000, Roc'nRollR (his then e-mail address) reluctantly took me to the airport for my flight back to California. Within the month I resumed my relationship with Michael and everything seemed to be getting back on track.

Three more busy years went by – traveling, house-renovating, working and living. One breast was slightly smaller and with a small scar but the cancer stayed away. I had regular yearly mammograms and nothing suspicious showed up. I was still lumpy but I felt no "activity."

4

That Knowing Feeling

The intuitive mind is a sacred gift and the rational mind is a faithful servant. We have created a society that honors the servant and has forgotten the gift.

–Albert Einstein

2003

In the spring of 2003 I felt a thickness and "something" in the area of the original cancer. I went to the Revlon Breast Center at UCLA and had an ultrasound. I met with a nurse practitioner there. The ultrasound did not show anything according to her and she said, after her clinical breast examination, "Everything is fine." The actual report reads: "No suspicious masses or areas of architecture distortion in either breast to suggest malignancy. Ultrasound identified normal breast tissue."

Again, let me remind you, we are talking about one of the best health care facilities in America. I was falsely relieved and believed the good news but went through the summer questioning the findings. I realize now I wasn't feeling well that summer – not sick, just fatigued and drained. I was also going through the trials of a romantic relationship that wasn't going well, which certainly didn't help, but I think physically I was being seriously challenged.

In early September of 2003 I had an appointment with my gynecologist, Dr. Paul Crane, in Beverly Hills for an annual check-up. I pointed out the thickness on my left breast that concerned me and he said he would like to biopsy it right there in the office. I was happy not to have to wait and make an appointment with a breast doctor and thought why not. So with help from his physician assistant he did an ultrasound guided biopsy and sent it off to the lab. A week or so later it came back with the all clear. I still wasn't convinced that I was fine but I wanted to believe the results – after all he sent it to a good lab.

The end of that month I split up with Michael, my long-time boyfriend – a 9-year mostly on-again, off-again relationship. I had to find a new place to live and think about what life was going to be like as a single woman in my mid-40s. It was a time full of transition and a mixture of sadness over the circumstances, relief that we had made a decision, and uncertainty about the future. Little did I know what lay ahead.

In October, as I was searching for a new place to live, I remember feeling fullness in the spot that had gotten thicker. I was living in Michael's Malibu beach house for a month and my dear friends from England, Pat and Gerry, were staying with me. It was beautiful outside, but my body kept on calling my attention back to my chest. "Damn, this still doesn't feel right." I made an appointment to go back to City of Hope.

In November 2003 I moved into a new house and I went back to Dr. Wagman, my oncology surgeon, at City of Hope, who suggested another mammogram. In early December I had another mammogram at City of Hope. When I left the appointment the radiologist thought everything looked fine and told me so. For the third time I was told by professionals that everything was fine, yet I still wasn't convinced. The report actually said, "No mammographic abnormality is seen in the area of patient concern in either breast." I insisted on an ultrasound and a biopsy. It was scheduled for early January 2004.

TIP: It is easy for months to go by between appointments, so discuss with your doctor what diagnostic procedures might be necessary and ask to have them scheduled together.

The Monday after Christmas 2003 my sister-in-law, Peggy Armenti, died in Michigan from renal cancer. I spent the last week of her life with her and watched her do battle. It takes so much bravery. Her body was swollen from the tumor, her skin was peeling off due to chemo and fluid retention and her mind was confused due to the drugs. The degeneration and circumstances made me so sad. How could someone look so healthy and then get so sick so quickly? Peggy was a former oncology nurse. She knew, better than most, what lay ahead and still she faced it with courage.

I remember at one point her husband, Fred, my brother and a surgeon, called during the day from the hospital to see how she was doing. I told her Fred was on the phone. In a morphine haze she said, "My Fred?" I told her, "Yes, your Fred." They had been married 25 years at this point. I handed her the phone. Disoriented from the drugs she put the phone to her heart rather than her ear. "Fred, Fred?" she called. From the chair where she spent the last weeks of her life she looked up at me childlike, frustrated. "I can't hear him." I raised the phone to her ear. It was heartbreaking.

That night the ambulance came to take her to the hospital. While her daughters knew the ambulance was coming, I didn't want them to have to see their mom leave the house that way, fairly certain she wasn't coming back home. I told them they should give their mom a hug and encouraged them to go out and get the Christmas tree with their friends. Peggy was 50 years old with a husband who loved her and took care of her and two of the most adorable girls in the world. She had everything to live for. All a grim reminder that there is no fairness when it comes to cancer, only reality.

TIP: Cancer happens to all kinds of people. No one group gets a pass, not even doctor's wives or rock star's wives (Linda McCartney) or for that matter rock stars (Sheryl Crow and Melissa Etheridge). It neither discriminates nor is it exclusive.

2004

In early January at City of Hope I had the ultrasound I insisted on even though the mammogram was clear. The ultrasound showed a mass so that same day I had the core biopsy that I thought should have been done in December. During the biopsy the radiologist again was not very sensitive to my pain. At one point he looked at me oddly, questioning me as to whether it really hurt or not. He was telling me about his kids and what a handful they were. I could not have cared less in my situation. He was wearing a yarmulke which had flipped and was dangling precariously off his head, held by a single bobby pin, and I anticipated it falling on me as he bent over my body. The biopsy gun went off several times. What he was doing hurt like hell. The female nurses in the room, aware that he wasn't acknowledging my distress, were very uncomfortable. I could see conflict registered on their faces. They shifted their weight from one leg to the other, resisting the urge to grab the gun and do it with more compassion. When he again questioned my pain, I finally asked him what he thought it would feel like if I took this same biopsy gun to his testicles. That got his attention.

TIP: Radiologists are trained at reading X-rays and in my experience many of them are not comfortable doing a biopsy. It should be done by someone who is skilled and unafraid of dealing with the human body, not just reading films. Make sure your radiologist is very experienced at doing the actual biopsy. And again, make certain you are given enough pain medicine before they start to work on

you. They have a schedule that they are trying to keep to but it is your body.

I waited a long week for my results from City of Hope. Dr. Wagman was traveling and no one else would give me the results over the phone: hospital policy. I called every day. It was very frustrating to have to wait, especially when I felt it wasn't going to be good news. Finally, the following week, the doctor called. It was malignant. My suspicions were confirmed. The third week of January 2004 I had another open biopsy (lumpectomy) at City of Hope.

TIP: If you are anxious about your results, set up ahead of time that the doctor or someone you designate will call you at home at the earliest possible time.

Michael took me to City of Hope and waited while I was being operated on. We had broken up months ago but he wanted to take me to the hospital. As I still hadn't told anyone else what was going on with me he was the obvious choice although it had a sad side as well. He picked me up at 5:30A.M. I remember being in the prep room before surgery, Michael sitting in a chair next to the bed. He had his hand under my lower back as I lay on the gurney, naked under the flimsy ugly hospital gown, hair net and all. I must have looked ravishing. The nurse was taking a medical history and recording the events. She said, "Husband by your side." I said, "No." She looked perplexed. He said, "Boyfriend." I said, "Former boyfriend." I remember the nurse looked at me funny. I am sure she was thinking, then what the heck is he doing here? What can I say except, relationships are complicated. Against hospital policy she let him stay. I remember he looked so happy that he was able to be there for me. Turns out this day was our last day together. Still I had been in that same pre-op room before alone and it was better, much better, to have him next to me.

The nurse had trouble inserting my IV and once in, it hurt. I tried to live with the ache, even putting ice on it, but finally asked them to redo it, which another nurse did. The pain went away. They don't like to be questioned and redo things but this falls under the category of, "Frankly my dear, I don't give a damn."

TIP: Your IV shouldn't hurt after it has been inserted. It means it either was not properly placed or is poorly seated and needs to be adjusted; you have a right to request that. It is not just a matter of comfort, but also one of safety.

In the recovery room, I slowly came out of the anesthetic-induced haze. I again experienced that underwater feeling. A new nurse then said, "Your husband is in the waiting room, I'll get him." The drugs make you so emotional and I was in tears trying to explain to her he wasn't my husband, he wasn't even my boyfriend. I felt so out of control, powerless and fragile; I just wanted to get the facts straight. I was so sad about the circumstances – that I was in the hospital again and while he was there today I was alone in this – the tears were hard to hold back.

We stopped on the way home and Michael picked up some take-out deli food as I hadn't been able to eat since the night before. The pain medicine made me really groggy. We got back to my house, lay down on my bed and took a nap together. Right before falling asleep, I put my hand on his chest, then I thought better of it and took it back. He took my hand and put it back on his chest, saying, "No leave it there." We fell asleep for two hours. We got up and he went out to get us some food. He came back with dinner and six bottles of wine – stocking my bar. I guess he thought I would be drinking a lot after this. He left at 10:00 P.M. and I went to bed. Other than a black tie event two months later where we were both in the crowd and one day at a stop sign, I didn't see him again for three years. This is the downside of having only one person in your circle of confidence: you really count on that person and feel the loss when he or she isn't there.

I was told after that surgery that they got it all. The tumor was 1.5 cm with clear margins and node negative. I was swollen but relieved that the cancer was gone, or so they told me. Over Super Bowl weekend I drove to Las Vegas with a friend. I wasn't fully recovered and the drive was really too much, but I wanted to escape and what better place to escape reality than Vegas? I bought a pair of Chanel black pants and very high-heel black shoes on sale that weekend. I still think of escape when I wear them. Pure escape.

In the winter of '04, on a ski trip to Vail, I told my friend Pam what had been going on with me. We are very close with, at that point, 30 years of friendship. She was shocked and hurt that I hadn't told her sooner. Of course at that time I thought I was fine and life was going to roll on like normal.

In March, when the swelling went down, I could feel a small nodule near the scar. I wasn't thinking it was cancer but I did think why the heck didn't the surgeon take it out when he had the chance? Reluctantly, forcing myself to look at it rather than look away, I made another appointment and went back to City of Hope to discuss it with Dr. Wagman.

That month I had my appointment with Dr. Wagman and also a consultation with an oncologist at City of Hope. During the meeting with the oncologist they advised me to have four rounds of chemotherapy. While the statistic for my survival was 70-75% for ten years without chemotherapy and 81% with chemotherapy it was suggested that I should have the treatment but was told it was my choice, considering my tumor was smaller than 2 centimeters and I was node negative. I was also encouraged to go on Tamoxifen. They gave me only survival statistics and not recurrence statistics.

During my appointment with Dr. Wagman I asked him if he would re-excise the spot and take out the nodule that was still apparent. He examined me, and said it was "normal breast tissue." He told me if I was worried I should have a mastectomy or he would just follow me with manual (clinical) examinations. I left that day feeling unsatisfied and powerless, wishing I could somehow remove it myself and not deal with unacceptable answers. Of course there was also a voice saying, "You're fine, be happy."

ESTROGEN BLOCKERS

Over 70% of breast cancers are hormone receptive. Drugs that are offered like tamoxifen (Nolvadex) for pre-menopausal women (estrogen blockers) and Arimidex (anastrozole) for post-menopausal women (estrogen stoppers) work by not allowing the estrogen to feed the cells. These estrogen blockers and stoppers have possible side effects such as more intense hot flashes, moodiness, possible early menopause, bone, joint and muscle pains, infertility, blood clots, bone loss and eye problems, and all can manifest, as well as cause other side effects, which you need to discuss with your doctor.

Many women take these drugs every day for a number of years. For example, a typical protocol for Tamoxifen is every day for five years. Many other women decide that the benefits do not outweigh the risks. It is important to get fully informed as to your individual benefit. It will be based on studies as they have no way of telling absolutely how these drugs will affect you but it is important to know what your options are. Be careful to fully evaluate the statistics as proponents have a tendency to frame them in such a way to make you think they are more effective than they are. For instance if a certain drug is 50% more effective at something but your chances of doing fine are already 80% without the drug, that 50% is not as much of a percentage

of survival as you might think. Just a caution to check the statistics and facts carefully.

AROMATASE INHIBITORS

Aromatase inhibitors can be used only for women who have hormone sensitive cancers. For women with estrogen positive tumors, blocking estrogen to the tumor becomes the goal. Estrogen is formulated in stages and it takes the enzyme aromatase to finalize this process. The drugs that are called "aromatase inhibitors" or (AIs) such as Arimidex, Aromasin and Femara are given to post-menopausal women to stop the production of estrogen. Faslodex is another drug that cements itself to the estrogen receptor and blocks its ability to act. Faslodex is injected monthly rather than taken in a daily pill form like the others. Again, there are side effects such as bone loss and other responses to these drugs that need to be discussed at length with your doctor before taking any medication.

HERCEPTIN or TYKERB

Herceptin was developed as a way to "turn off" the HER2/neu gene. It is an antibody to the HER2/neu protein. If you are HER2/neu positive this may be a treatment for you. Tykerb is also sometimes used when there is too much HER2/neu protein.

TRIPLE NEGATIVE

A triple negative diagnosis means you are ER and PR negative and are also HER2/neu negative. This would indicate your kind of cancer is not hormone receptive and in addition you would also not be a candidate for Herceptin or Tykerb. Surgery, radiation and/or chemotherapy are the standard therapy for a triple negative diagnosis. The need for early diagnosis is especially vital given the aggressive nature of this type of breast cancer.

5

Facing What I Was Avoiding

Once I allowed the real possibility of a mastectomy to enter my consciousness, life as I knew it ended.

–Jessica Queller, *Pretty is what Changes*

For two months the nodule didn't grow but it didn't go away either. Every time I touched it I felt as if it "should" come out. I wasn't satisfied with the diagnosis of "normal breast tissue" and a month later went to see Dr. Jerrold Steiner, at Cedars-Sinai Medical Center, the doctor who found the original abnormal cells. He agreed to take it out and take a look at it.

Pam flew out from New Jersey to be with me for the surgery. I picked her up in Long Beach and took her straight to a birthday party for some other girlfriends – nicknamed my "goddess friends." It is always fun to have your friends from different areas of your life meet, especially when they have heard so much about one another. It was a light-hearted evening for everyone else and I tried not to think about the next day.

June 20, 2004. When we arrived at the Breast Center at Cedars-Sinai Medical Center in Beverly Hills I asked Pam to come into the bathroom with me. "Here, I want to show you before they take it out." She had had her own run in with DCIS and knew all too well the fear and uncertainty surrounding breast cancer. I knew she was thinking it was a small nodule, and the surgeons were just in there, so it must be okay, but she looked worried. Maybe it was my reflection I saw in her face. Before I went into surgery I made an appointment for her to get her hair cut at Jose Eber in Beverly Hills with my hairdresser – someone should have great hair today. There is no chance it will be me underneath those awful surgery caps. The surgery (lumpectomy) was uneventful but tiring, and we went home and waited.

On Monday the surgeon called me. It turned out to be malignant again. I went in to see Dr. Steiner that week and he said two things at that point, "You probably saved your life and you have to have a mastectomy." What I had been avoiding for years was now an inevitable outcome...losing my breast.

I wonder now if I had had the chemotherapy and gone on tamoxifen that March, as recommended by City of Hope, the nodule would have diminished to the degree that I wouldn't have seen it and therefore not had it excised? Would that have allowed the cancer to grow undetected? We will never know.

In the middle of this another issue more and more patients are faced with arose – having their doctor opt out of their insurance plan. Dr. Steiner decided not to take Blue Cross insurance anymore so I either needed to pay him cash or find a new surgeon who would take my insurance. As it turns out even the lumpectomy cost $3,000 because he was no longer a "provider."

TIP: "Provider" means that the doctor and/or hospital are part of your insurance company's system (in-network). If they aren't a "provider" there may be an "out-of-network" fee they offer but more often than not you will have to negotiate their fee directly.

"Recurrence" is the scariest word next to cancer and what everyone who has been through a cancer diagnosis dreads. When you face breast cancer the first time you may think, okay, I can beat this, but when it comes back again you learn not to underestimate your opponent. And you have more knowledge as to the energy, resources and strength needed to engage. Just the knowing alone can be draining. Any illusion that this is going to be simple has long since become a fantasy and you are left with the feeling that once again you have to muster the courage and will to fight this battle. You can't hide. That's a tempting but unacceptable alternative. You must face it.

According to the statistics, most breast cancers recur, if they are going to recur, within the first three years. Of course, my case proves the exception. My breast cancer was definitively diagnosed in 1999 (although in 1996 doctors found abnormal cells in the same area and I think missed the cancer). My recurrence wasn't detected until 2003. So again, while there are statistics you may very well be the exception.

In my case, I always felt it was more like they had misdiagnosed it in 1996 and missed getting all of it in 1999, the first time I had a set of lumpectomies. I didn't see it so much as a recurrence as a continued growth of something they left behind. Now that I have had a mastectomy and have been "cleaned out," a recurrence would make me feel as though I can't beat it: like trick candles on a birthday cake that continually relight. All the blowing in the world won't make it go away. This isn't necessarily true, but it is how I would feel.

So given the frightening nature of a recurrence it is important to be aware of some of the actual symptoms if it were to recur. If you experience any of these symptoms see your physician immediately. Recurrence can either be local (in the breast of the original cancer) or distant (away from the breast area). If it were to show up in the other breast it would be considered a new cancer.

LOCAL RECURRENCE

A thickening or lump in the area of the original cancer. This often happens along the scar or skin near the site but not always. Some women worry that reconstruction implants

would make a recurrence hard to identify, especially since mammography is not often used to monitor when there is an implant after reconstruction for fear of rupturing the implant. If this concerns you, you should discuss it with your doctor. A lot would depend on where your original cancer was located.

REGIONAL RECURRENCE

A swelling of the lymph nodes would indicate there may be a regional recurrence. The swelling could be under your arm, at the center of your chest along the sternum or around your collarbone.

DISTANT RECURRENCE

Constant and continuing pain that cannot be attributed to arthritis or some other medical condition may indicate a distant recurrence. This is of course the symptom that makes every ache and pain a source of concern. Bone pain you cannot dismiss.

A persistent (over a week) headache that doesn't go away.

Shortness of breath or a cough that is persistent even when treated and not attributed to a cold.

Unexplained weight loss.

Again, all recurrences, like all breast cancers, are not alike. If the recurrence is in the same local area perhaps it can be treated as the first occurrence was with surgery and/or radiation and/or chemotherapy, depending on whether you had radiation and/or chemotherapy the first time and if there is node involvement. There is a limit to how much overall radiation or chemotherapy a person can

tolerate so these are factors in deciding what to do next. If the recurrence is distant then the disease has metastasized and the treatment plan would almost certainly include chemotherapy. It could also include radiation to shrink the tumor at the new site and perhaps more surgery as well.

Some of the factors that would affect the chances of a recurrence are the pathology of the cancer, tumor size, lymph node involvement, and tumor markers. But nothing can determine for sure if you will have a recurrence. We are talking odds here, not certainty.

FACTORS THAT IMPACT RECURRENCE

Women who are node positive are more likely to have a recurrence. The more nodes that were positive the higher your chances are of a recurrence.

The grade of the tumor.
The lower the grade the less chance of a recurrence. The grade measures the amount of normal cells in the tumor.

Cell growth rate.
Slower growth is related to less chance of recurrence.

Hormone receptor.
Positive HR is lower risk than Negative HR.

Size of the tumor.
The smaller the tumor, the lower the risk.

Knowing I had to have a mastectomy, my sadness that July was palpable. A friend suggested we go to a dude ranch, Rock Springs, in Oregon with her kids and another girlfriend and her daughter, for a few days. It was a breath of fresh air that helped get me through the next couple of months.

I love being around animals, particularly horses and dogs, and horseback riding that summer with views of the Twin Sister Mountains and Mt. Bachelor is a great memory to this day. I used to jump horses and compete as a kid and riding a horse is like riding a bike for me. I am instantly balanced and at home. Still, I was a bit swollen from the surgery and my underarm hurt. Was that the cancer? Was there an infection? My arm was swollen and numb. Was it the plane ride? Or is more going on? That is the insidious nature of cancer, it keeps you constantly guessing. Around the horses and my friends, kayaking on Spark Lake and cantering through the acres of government land, there were moments of freedom when I forgot what was ahead of me. But I knew I had to have this surgery and soon. I was glad to be there but also anxious to get back to L.A. and get this done.

It was clear to me that I would want to do some sort of reconstruction simultaneously so the next step was to look for a team of surgeons to do the operation. If you do it simultaneously then both of your surgeons, an oncology surgeon and a plastic surgeon, need to be available and have privileges at the same hospital. Finding a team you like isn't always easy.

TIP: Reconstruction is a way for a woman to feel somewhat restored but some opt not to have more surgery. Again this is an individual choice. Reconstruction can happen at the time of the mastectomy or at a later date. There are a number of factors that need to be considered, including but not limited to what kind of surgery you are suited for (for instance a tram flap requires that there be enough tissue at the host site), expense, period of recovery, end result you are willing to live with, and the expertise of your plastic surgeon.

I made the rounds. I saw some of the best plastic surgeons in Beverly Hills for consultations. Dr. Slate, Dr. Tearston, Dr. Orringer, Dr. D., Dr. Da Lio. Not one of them, by the way, was satisfied with only my Blue Cross insurance and required I pay additional cash. Even though by law breast reconstruction must be covered by insurance, the amount insurance reimburses is not sufficient for them. So if you want their work you pay with cash on top of the insurance reimbursement.

At that point I wanted Dr. Steiner, who was at the Breast Center at Cedars- Sinai Medical Center, to do the cancer removal part of the surgery so I arranged to meet with Dr. R. Kendrick Slate, a plastic surgeon, who also had privileges at Cedars-Sinai Medical Center. The day of my appointment he had on cowboy boots (not typical footwear in L.A.). and expressed himself in a very straight forward manner. At his hospital office he spent two hours patiently explaining all the procedures to me. As he was describing the tunnel tram flap procedure I nearly fainted. This is a procedure where skin and muscle are taken from your stomach and then tunneled under your mid-section and repositioned as a breast. Not only did I have cancer again, and I was going to lose my breast, I may end up with a huge scar across my stomach and they may have to tunnel a flap of skin under my stomach muscles to my breast area. I left there with my head spinning and thinking there must be a better way. The advantages of this surgery are the newly formed mound is your own tissue and therefore will be warm, will move more like your natural breast and will lose and gain weight with the rest of your body. The disadvantages from my point of view are a much longer recovery – at least 6 weeks, numbness at the host site, and a huge scar across my stomach.

TIP: Tram surgery needs adequate tissue at the host site and on thinner women it isn't always optimal or even possible.

A few days later I went to see another plastic surgeon who is affiliated with Cedars-Sinai Medical Center, Dr. Gary Tearston. As I sat on the examining table and explained my history I started to cry. I had been fairly composed up to this point but I guess retelling the story once again just overwhelmed me. It was as though I was crying for someone else. Dr. Tearston is Stanford trained and his presentation and demeanor was very efficient, as professional as his office brochure. He rolled over a tray of implants like desserts at a fancy restaurant and said he would do some sort of combination of skin and implant. He seemed well qualified to do the surgery. The cost loomed, $12,000, first payment with a check written upfront to Cedars just to get in the door. Why does this have to cost so much on top of my insurance?

From there I went to see Dr. D., (not his real initial) a Beverly Hills plastic surgeon. He was part of my investigation to find a plastic surgeon in Beverly Hills that could do the reconstruction and had privileges at Cedars. What is important is that they not only have privileges at the same hospital but hopefully some experience working together.

His office was immaculate and beautiful – everything you want from a plastic surgery office including being asked to wear booties when you go to the patient area to be examined. I could tell he was a compulsive perfectionist. I remember Dr. D. looked at my breasts and said, "Are you sure you want to do this?" He is my age, and I did for a second feel like I was on a date. He looked as sad as me. Not wanting to be reminded how hard this is going to be I said, "Yes, I don't think I have a choice." Cancer isn't the common reason people seek out plastic surgeons, especially Beverly Hills plastic surgeons, but I wasn't there for a nose job. No, this was serious and not optional and the consequences weren't good. At this point I was getting pain in my left breast; I knew it had to come off. He advised me against the implant procedure that I thought I wanted and recommended Dr. Jay Orringer, another Beverly Hills plastic surgeon, who is a specialist in a flap procedure.

I made the appointment with Dr. Orringer. His office was in the penthouse and slick enough you would have expected them to film scenes from HBO's "Entourage" there. He was professional, in a crisp white lab coat, and was the only doctor who actually measured me. He discussed the tram flap procedure or having a lattisimus dorsi flap procedure – where tissue from your back is moved to your breast. It sounded horrific to me. Again the cost seemed outrageous given I had insurance.

I then considered using a plastic surgeon at St. John's Hospital in Santa Monica but in that case I would need an oncology surgeon who had privileges there. Dr. Armando Giuliano, an oncology surgeon, was recommended to me. His waiting room looked like your grandmother's house – chintz fabric and oak furniture. His female physician assistant examined me. Then he came in, looked at me, looked at my chart and said, "You're young…we will be very aggressive with you." It was clear he had done this thousands of times. Still it didn't feel right.

On June 24, 2004, I went to UCLA, where I thought I might have the surgery. I met with Dr. Helen Chang, the oncology surgeon from the Revlon Breast Center, whom I liked very much. She has a wonderful reputation but I am not a big fan of the Breast Center at UCLA. I had gone there for a second opinion, which they conducted partially in a group clinic setting that I found very uncomfortable. Plus they had been wrong about my ultrasound a year earlier.

For me, so much of the decision-making process is about who gives you the most confidence. While I liked Dr. Chang, I found the UCLA Breast Center's processes to be disconnected from the doctors, often using nurse practitioners and I just didn't like the way they set-up appointments. I knew I was going to be rather alone in this phase and I needed a more hands-on, personal approach. Still, for a few days, I thought this was going to be my path so I went to UCLA to have the pre-op tests and made an appointment to see a plastic surgeon there.

TIP: There are pre-operative tests that you must have done prior to surgery. Blood work, an EKG and a chest X-ray are usually the minimum that is required and others, like a bone scan, may be required as well. If for some reason you are physically far away from where you are having the surgery it may be possible for you to have this standard pre-op work done elsewhere and have the results faxed or e-mailed to the hospital where the surgery is scheduled.

WHAT IS AN EKG?

An EKG is an electrocardiogram. It records the electrical activity of the heart. Depending on your age and overall fitness, doctors like to have a baseline tracing of your heart's rate and rhythm. They will put pads on you with wires that are hooked up to a small machine. It is a painless and non-invasive test.

WHAT IS A CHEST X-RAY?

A chest X-ray is a radiograph of the chest and provides information about your heart silhouette, your lungs, the contour of your diaphragm and mediastinal structures.

WHAT IS A BONE SCAN?

A bone scan is used to evaluate changes in the bone in order to detect if the cancer has spread (metastasized) to the bones. They are also used to evaluate conditions that can affect the bone such as trauma or infection. A bone scan can sometimes detect a problem much earlier than a regular X-ray. It is a test that can be conducted on the entire body or just a particular part. The bone scan is administered by injecting a tracer (radioactive material) into the vein which travels though the bloodstream and into the bones. It takes 1-3 hours for the tracer to be picked up by the scanner. Areas of rapid bone growth absorb more

radioactive material and show up as white or "hot spots." Areas that show up as dark may indicate a lack of blood supply to the bone. Other than the injection site, the bone scan should be painless.

WHAT IS A MASTECTOMY?

A mastectomy is a surgery where the goal is to remove all the breast tissue. Sometimes the surgeon will have to include lymph nodes and muscle depending on the location and size of the tumor. The decision to have a single mastectomy (one breast) or a double mastectomy (both breasts) depends on your diagnosis and sometimes on your personal preference. A double mastectomy will likely give you a more symmetrical result but some women do not want to have surgery on a breast that isn't showing any signs of disease and opt for a single mastectomy.

There is SIMPLE MASTECTOMY which is the removal of the entire breast but not the lymph nodes or the muscle.

MODIFIED RADICAL MASTECTOMY is the removal of the breast and some of the lymph nodes. (This is the most common, and the surgery that I had.)

And RADICAL MASTECTOMY is the removal of the breast, all of the lymph nodes, and the muscle underneath the breast. This is not as common anymore but necessary if the tumor is located on the chest wall.

Even in a MODIFIED RADICAL MASTECTOMY the surgeon tries to remove all the breast tissue – ducts, lobes, fat, everything. Most times the nipple is also removed but occasionally, depending on the diagnosis, the nipple can be spared. The general goal here is to remove all the

breast tissue so the breast cancer has nowhere to grow. And while this is the goal, there is no way for a surgeon to be sure they have removed every speck of breast tissue. With a mastectomy there is a substantial amount of swelling and drains are often inserted temporarily to help remove the fluid that builds up after surgery. There is usually an attempt to save as much skin as possible to facilitate any reconstruction procedure.

IS RECONSTRUCTION RIGHT FOR YOU?

Not everyone has reconstruction and again this is an individual choice. If you decide that you are *not* going to have breast reconstruction you may opt for a prosthesis, which you insert into your bra, instead of more surgery. A prosthesis can give you more symmetry with a bra, in terms of weight and appearance, and that may be sufficient for you.

If you do decide to opt for a prosthesis there are several companies that offer prosthetic devices and some are listed in the resource guide at the back of this book. For some the cost and the thought of more surgery may be enough to make you decide not to have reconstruction. Other women don't like the idea of something foreign, like an implant, in their bodies. And some women are so consumed with fighting the disease that reconstruction isn't on their priority list.

I knew I would have reconstruction and that impacted my decisions. However, I didn't know what that entailed or how best to accomplish it. I didn't know anyone who had gone through the process so I didn't have anyone to ask what to expect. And I didn't know what it would feel like on that side without any breast tissue, or how radiated tissue reacts differently to an implant or how to be clear with the doctors about what my expectations of the reduction side should look like so that I could have the symmetry I was seeking.

While I was at UCLA to get blood work, an EKG and a chest X-ray, I noticed I was hardly breathing. Hospitals have that effect on me. I can feel anxiety bubble up and I know I am not alone in this reaction. For many people just being inside the walls of a hospital can generate anxiety – something health care workers don't quite appreciate.

I used to say to my former boyfriend, who is an avid photographer and was constantly taking pictures of me, that I was the most photographed woman in Los Angeles. Now I really feel like that is true. Bone scans, chest X-ray, PET scan, breast MRIs, ultrasounds and mammograms – there isn't an inch of me that hasn't been documented. It is hard to feel whole when it is the parts that are constantly being scrutinized.

HOW WILL IT BE DECIDED IF YOU NEED CHEMOTHERAPY?

The decision whether or not to have chemotherapy can be a complicated one especially if it is *not* detected in your lymph nodes. Often the assumption is made that if it has not traveled beyond the breast, the tumor is less than 2 centimeters and you are Node Negative, chemotherapy is not automatic. If you are Node Positive they will remove the affected nodes plus a few more and generally give you chemotherapy in order to kill any microscopic cells that have ventured beyond those lymph nodes. If the tumor is large than they may give you chemotherapy first to shrink the tumor before surgery.

WHAT IS A TRAM FLAP?

The TRAM flap uses the lower abdominal muscle, skin and tissue. Sometimes this is also known as the "tummy tuck"

method of reconstruction. This ellipse of an area, if still attached, is rotated and then tunneled under the stomach area and positioned at the breast area.

It can also be done in a "free flap" way, but this takes even more expertise and microsurgery. The advantage of this procedure is that it is your own tissue in place of the breast. The new breast area will gain and lose weight with the rest of you and it shouldn't need to be redone. The disadvantage is that it is a much more expensive and involved procedure with a longer recovery time. And the host site will likely have some weakness and certainly some numbness.

WHAT IS A DIEP FLAP?

A DIEP flap is similar to the TRAM in that the same lower abdominal area is involved but the surgeon does not take the muscle and therefore leaves less chance of weakness in the host area. This is a free flap, meaning at one point it is completely detached from the body before being reattached with microsurgery. It is important that the blood supply, which is reattached using microsurgery, succeeds; otherwise the flap will fail and further surgery will be necessary. Again your surgeon would require a large degree of expertise to be competent in this kind of procedure.

WHAT IS A LATTISIMUS DORSI FLAP?

The Lattisimus Dorsi Flap procedure uses the lattisimus dorsi muscle from the side of your back. If you were to serve a tennis ball this is the muscle that would be fully engaged. To get the proper size and dimension of the breast an implant is often used together with the muscle. There may be some loss of function and certainly numbness in the host area. And it could affect your range of motion on that side.

WHAT IS A GLUT FLAP?

Another possibility is the Gluteal Free Flap which uses tissue, skin and muscle taken from the buttock area – either from the superior (top) or inferior (bottom) location. These are free flaps and require a high level of expertise and skill in microsurgery. Taking tissue from this area can leave the area asymmetrical unless done on both sides in the case of a double reconstruction.

I met with Dr. Andrew Da Lio, a UCLA plastic surgeon, who would be the plastic surgeon if I chose Dr. Chang as my oncology surgeon. A friend of mine, Nancy, came to the appointment with me and as he walked in I could see her eyes light up – he was handsome. We exchanged greetings and he was not there two minutes before I whipped off my shirt so he could examine my breasts. My friend was surprised at my lack of modesty, but I am here for answers and the sooner he examines me the sooner we can start discussing what he is capable of doing for me. Experience has taught me that surgeons have short attention spans and limited time so I want to cut to the chase. He was attractive and it could be worse waking up from surgery to see his face but his suggestion of the tram flap procedure freaked me out again.

TIP: If you are having tram reconstruction you won't be able to reach for much or move anything heavy around. Make sure everything is within reach and anything heavy you may need is in a certain position before you go into the hospital.

That night I decided I wanted to do the surgery with just an implant and not a tram flap. I realized as much as having my own tissue as a breast mound would be desirable, I didn't want to be numb across my stomach, have another scar and a long recovery. I decided that I would try an implant and if it didn't work out I could always have the more complicated procedure of a tram flap later.

On the 26th of July, 2004, I phoned my brother Fred, a cardiothoracic surgeon and Chief of Surgery at McLaren Regional Medical Center in Michigan. I explained to him how I was having a hard time finding a team I was comfortable with in Los Angeles. Ironic really, as you would think in Los Angeles, a Mecca when it comes to fake breasts, finding a team would have been as easy as a Laker slam-dunk. But of course there was more going on. The universe was not supplying what was not to be.

Fred told me again that I could go there and have the whole thing done in Michigan. He gave me the name of a plastic surgeon he works with in Flint, Dr. Abd Alghanem. I didn't know if my insurance would cover me in another state, so I hadn't previously considered this seriously and I was reluctant to put his daughters though more cancer trauma but, I said I would call the plastic surgeon. Was it coincidental that I had already met the oncology surgeon if I went to Michigan, Dr. Kamal Saha the previous December? His lovely wife, Luci, was my sister-in-law's best friend and Fred had already told me what a good surgeon he was, so in a way I had already been given one piece of the puzzle before the purpose became apparent.

TIP: Consider having the procedure in another state if you have support there and if you can find a team that will take your insurance. You must call the insurance company in advance and make certain they will cover you. It may be much cheaper in the long run and better for your recovery if you can go where your support system is the best.

July 27, 2004. I talk to Dr. Alghanem, the plastic surgeon in Michigan. I was explaining everything that had gone on and at this point I was like a professional patient and rattling off dates, doctors and disappointments with proficiency. When I finished there was silence on the other end of the phone. "Are you still there?" I asked. Usually the surgeons pepper you with questions. I wasn't accustomed to the quiet. "Yes, I'm listening." He sounded very calm and reassuring. I had one last question for him. I asked him if he was going to be in town and if he was sure he could fit me into his schedule. I didn't want to go to Michigan and wait. He said, "For Fred I will do it Sunday at midnight." Suddenly it all became clear. If my insurance company would cover it I would go to Michigan. I called my insurance and, lo and behold, they said they would cover me. I flew out the next day. I was terrified of what was ahead but very grateful to have a doctor in the family.

July 28, 2004. Tuesday I took the red eye to Michigan with my dog, Cinder. Wednesday Fred took me to meet with Dr. Alghanem. He examined me and we talked about using an expander and implant. The expander is a sort of place-holder implant that is put in first to expand the tissue and muscle. He agreed that this could give me a good result and that I didn't need to have the more elaborate tram procedure. I saw Dr. Saha, the oncology surgeon, and met with him and his associate to discuss the surgery and how I was feeling.

July 29, 2004. I scheduled everything. Had a breast MRI – 6,000 images of my breasts. I asked the radiologist if I could see it. Clearly, it again confirmed the breast cancer.

TIP: If you have an MRI and are the least bit claustrophobic, bring with you one of those heavy eye masks for sleeping. The ones with some weight to them are better. If you put this on *before* you go into the machine it may relieve your feelings of claustrophobia and help you get through the procedure. Even a "doughnut hole" machine (one with an open end) can be overwhelming to someone who is claustrophobic.

There are MRIs with and without contrast (the dye). Contrast delivers a more defined image, but it will require you to have an IV inserted.

July 30, 2004. I met with Dr. Maden Arora, an oncologist, Dr. Alghanem, the plastic surgeon, for another discussion and then with Dr. Saha, the oncology surgeon, for an exam. I went to the hospital and got the pre-admission paperwork done. It was there I filled out a hospital directive – "A Durable Power of Attorney for Health Care," which is a sobering but necessary document.

TIP: Give some thought to the "Hospital or Advance Directive" before this day arrives. The "Hospital Directive" spells out what your wishes are and who would make medical decisions for you if you are unable to do so yourself. It will designate a legal advocate in the event you are incapacitated and cannot participate in your medical treatment.

August 1, 2004. My surgery is scheduled for 10:30 A.M. Saturday morning. I am certainly scared about what is ahead of me. I went to McLaren Medical alone and checked in. Even though it was Saturday, Fred's already at the hospital doing surgery so I am in the reception area by myself. After a few questions from the nurses, I undress and put on the gown, and am up on the gurney and sedated.

This crisis seemed to put everything on the table for review. As I close my eyes I start to think about what I want to do when this is over. What would be fun, fulfilling, make me happy, comforting? Who will be in my life? Who will I let in? Will I get married again? (Yes, I really did ask myself that question.) Where do I want to travel? Where do I want to live? And the most pressing question, what will it be like to live without the body I have always known? I was unconscious before any answers appeared.

TIP: Wear something comfortable to the hospital that will be easy for you to put on when you leave the hospital: not something you pull over your head. I had a red cotton

hoodie (important to have a zipper front) with pockets and matching pants with an elastic waist. Comfortable, easy to put on and take off, washable and colorful. This is not the time to wear "old" clothes. Buy yourself something you feel good in with a little extra room and that is light-weight enough that it would be comfortable if you fell asleep in it. Also a good gift for anyone facing this kind of surgery.

After the four-hour surgery, as I was coming out of the anesthesia, I knew something was wrong. I dislike that state of uncontrolled emotional vulnerability as you awaken to the world, and the feeling of being submerged, but this time I was also having a hard time swallowing and I was getting waves of a strange sensation going up my arms and around my neck and head. I could not take a full breath and anticipated my air being completely cut off. I remember asking for my brother in a panic and then seeing his face over me as I came to.

What no one knew at the time was that I was having an allergic reaction to latex, which is what surgical gloves are made of. It was running through my system and every breath became questionable. I came out of the surgery at around 4:00 P.M. and was moved to a regular room but I was fighting for air as the soft tissue in the back of my throat swelled. The allergic reaction was over taking my system and all I wanted to do was down water to keep my throat open. Fred sat with me until 11:00 P.M. that evening. I drank four large bottles of Evian. My throat was constricting in a dangerous way and Fred noticed that my voice grew deeper as the reaction waved through my system, the swelling having an effect on my voice box. I just prayed that it wouldn't settle completely in my throat and cut off my air. They had given me a heavy dose of Benadryl, for the reaction, so between that and the earlier sedation I was in and out of consciousness. Large hives formed on my arms and back and I had to sit up, due to the surgery and my throat constricting.

At 11:00 P.M. Fred decided I needed to continue to be watched and had the nurses take me to the Intensive Care Unit. I was still in a very fuzzy state but I remember the noise of the machines and the yellow glow of the lights in my room. The nurses put a heart monitor on me and left me alone. I thought that will be just perfect, my throat will close, I will gasp for air, my heart will stop and then they will come and see what's wrong. I'll die not from the cancer but from the allergic reaction to the surgery. I slept only a half an hour at a time and each time I woke up I thought, "That's good; at least I'm still breathing."

TIP: If you suspect you are allergic to anything, especially latex, check it out with an allergist before you go into the hospital. A latex allergy can build up in your system so you can go from being asymptomatic to all of a sudden having a reaction. If you have had any chemical sensitivities or hives in the past this may be an indicator that you are at risk and it would be best to be seen by an allergist before surgery. Also if there is a family history of chemical sensitivity.

I am allergic to latex, which can be fatal. Not knowing this they operated on me with latex gloves, overdosing my organs with contact. If you have an allergic reaction histamine will release and overload your system. The soft tissue in your throat swells, closing the passageway and you can't get any air. You could go into what is called anaphylactic shock. This can happen if you are allergic to bee stings or peanuts and sundry other things. My only small clue that I had an allergy was a mild allergic reaction at the dentist about three months prior when the technician took X-rays and used latex gloves. A hive formed on my arm while I was in the dentist chair and that night my throat was tighter than normal. But never having had anything like that before I didn't connect it to latex gloves and didn't think to get tested for something specific. I should have. Luckily, the night of the surgery, I had someone watching me who could monitor and medicate me properly. The allergic reaction subsided but lasted four days and came in waves. It was certainly more immediately life-threatening than the cancer. Finally the doctors gave me a combination of drugs to get my body to stop reacting.

LATEX ALLERGY

Latex allergy has become a huge issue in American hospitals. The proliferation and long-time use of latex throughout medicine for everything from heart monitors to gloves makes anyone who is sensitive at risk. There has been a movement in the medical community away from the use of latex but its performance qualities of tight fit and thinness makes it perfect for surgery and they remain the gloves of choice. Had it been clear that I had a latex allergy the doctors would have made the surgery room a "latex free zone," including making me the first surgery of the day so there weren't any traces of latex powder in the air. But they had no way of knowing because I didn't know.

Owing to an increase in the number of patients with a latex sensitivity, hospitals are slowly making more and more equipment and areas latex free zones. But this is not something you can assume and even if the allergy is noted on your chart you still need to advise anyone who comes in contact with you while in a medical facility that you have a latex allergy, including emergency personnel. Of course any allergy, including food allergies, needs to be disclosed to hospital staff. Also if you have a latex allergy make sure your food is not being prepared with latex gloves at a hospital or restaurant. That kind of contact with something you ingest can surely bring on a reaction.

August 2, 2004. On Sunday Dr. Alghanem came by my hospital room to change the bandages and check the incision. I knew as soon as I saw him walk into my room, I was going to have to face my new body. As he was removing the bandages he tried to warn me that it wouldn't be like this forever, but the site made me cry. Instead of a beautiful breast I now had two pieces of skin stitched together, the nipple and the roundness gone. It was about an inch off my chest due to the expander but flat. It was horrible, no doubt about it. I think he felt bad that I was there without a husband or partner to comfort me. He also knew that I was away from my home and my friends. My brother and the girls were there, thank God, but it was pretty lonely.

Four women from the hospital auxiliary came in to see me that Sunday morning. They stood at the end of the bed and brought me a pink handmade pillow. It was U-shaped so it could be placed under my arm to relieve the pressure. I found out they gave them to all the breast cancer patients. The nurse was late giving me my pain medicine that morning and I was in no mood for visitors – especially strangers, even well-intentioned ones. I remember saying that morning I didn't need a "f&★% pink pillow," I needed Vicodin and I remember I wasn't nice about it. I felt like I was Debra Winger *and* Shirley MacLaine from *Terms of Endearment* all rolled into one. Of course, now when I look at that pillow I think of all the kindness that came my way during that time, but back then I was in too much pain, over the edge emotionally and physically – to be courteous.

And, as if I needed to be reminded that the universe has quite a sense of timing and irony, the flowers arrived, again. I should explain. As I was coming out of the surgery the night before and literally fighting for every breath, three dozen beautiful roses arrived. I suspected, before even looking at the card, that they were from Michael, my former boyfriend. I hadn't been in touch with him for months but the fact that he found out I was in the hospital did not surprise me. Just because you aren't together anymore doesn't always mean you are done; some relationships have an afterlife.

The flowers, while a lovely gesture, were just another searing reminder of the loneliness of this part of the crisis. When it was decided I needed to go to the ICU Saturday night the nurse asked me what I wanted to do with the flowers (flowers are not allowed in ICU). I said, "I don't care." The incredulous nurse asked, "You sure? They're beautiful. You sure you don't want them?" "Yes, I'm sure." She then said, "What should we do with them?" With more important things on my plate as I just had major breast surgery, my throat was closing and I was having trouble swallowing and breathing, I said, "Really, I don't care, give them away." She carried them out of the room shaking her head. I'm sure she was thinking "crazy woman from California."

When they took me up to the ICU that night for observation I thought for sure the flowers were ancient history but some things are just meant to be and sure enough the next day when they brought me back to the regular floor a new smiling nurse once again came in my room with the roses. "These came for you." I couldn't believe someone hadn't taken them home the night before. I looked at my brother, who was there when I sent them away and who knew more about the emotional trigger of the flowers. He looked at me and said, in the way only an older, protective brother can, a funny remark about the "boomerang" flowers. I let her put them on the table and there they sat for two more days.

Monday, August 3, 2004. At 7:00 A.M. Fred glided into my room full of purpose and energy. He looked so...healthy. It was a quick visit before his surgery day started. He held a bag with the bottled water I requested as I couldn't drink the hospital water and water was all I had a thirst for. I was in bed and crying. "What's wrong? You in pain?" he questioned as a doctor would. I wasn't, the strong pain meds had kicked in. "It's been... eleven years," was all I could manage though the sobs. Confused he said, "What?" "It's been... eleven years since Dad died. Today. Eleven years ago today." He nodded, not really knowing how to comfort me and surely wondering why I would go to such a place given the circumstances. Maybe he didn't realize that, because of who I am and the added psychological lubricant of the depressing drugs I had no choice. I was emotionally open like a smashed melon. I was in pieces...literally.

Suddenly life's losses seemed overwhelming. The sadness of losing my breast and having to deal with the cancer begot more sadness. Fact is, I missed my Dad especially in times like this. I knew if he were here his eyes would have been honestly sad but his words would have been encouraging. Like many other days when I felt bad growing up, he would assure me, "It's going to be okay." That was what I was longing for. These were dark days. I missed his light, his humor and protection. I left the hospital that Monday afternoon. Little did I know I would be back soon, and in the same room.

NOTE: If you are a hospital administrator *please* make the water in your hospital drinkable. Water is what most patients drink while in the hospital and it should be the best filtered water available.

The pain of the mastectomy was barely manageable with Vicodin and sleep came only with Ambien. I was told to keep a detailed chart of pain medicine, temperature, sleeping pills and how much fluid was draining. The expander was excruciatingly uncomfortable. It was as if ballpoint pen were sitting on my raw chest wall with a water balloon on top and a vice holding it in place. I felt like a foot was pressing on my chest all the time, the pressure was physically breath taking. My chest muscle, knowing where it was supposed to be, was continually trying to make its way back to where it has always been but the implant was in its path. My body, of course, was just trying to heal and get back to "normal." I was still having an allergic reaction, which was frightening, as my throat swelled in waves making me feel like my air was going to be cut off any second and I was having a hard time sleeping and getting comfortable. I could sleep only on my back, upright with a sleeping pill. I had a drain coming out of my body into a bulb like device called a Jackson Pratt drain. All I could think of was take this one minute at a time.

At my brother's house I slept most of the time and lay on the couch the rest. I was so uncomfortable with constant pressure and pain. I later found out it wasn't so much the expander but the drain under the expander that was unbearable. The drain customarily stays in for 10 to 14 days. Mine, due to the fact that it continued to drain, was in for seven weeks. It never stopped draining and the doctor finally had to just take it out and let my body equalize itself. Now I know why it is called a drain. It drains you of all energy. When you have an open wound (a drain opening) your body is using all its energy to close it and fight off infection. There was nothing left for anything else.

TIP: When you tell others you have an implant or implants sometimes people think it is like breast augmentation. The implant can be the same device but with a mastectomy there isn't any breast tissue left to cushion it so it doesn't feel the same as an augmentation and your chest wall is initially raw under the implant. Generally surgeons use the technique of placing the implant sub-muscular. The muscle covers the implant and on top of that is just skin so the implant is more apparent.

It was tough getting used to my new unbalanced body fully knowing I had to have more surgery to get closer to something that looked somewhat normal. The mirror was the enemy. It occurred to me that when someone dies in the Jewish religion the family covers the mirrors, as death is no time for vanity. This felt like a death. Maybe I should have covered the mirrors?

On Wednesday I found out that while the cancer was in more than one place in my breast – multicentric – and not good news, the other 8 lymph nodes that were removed and the bone marrow test were clear. I know that was *really good news* but I was so tired it didn't have much of an effect. The visiting nurse came to the house a number of times. She was helpful and tried to be jolly. It was pretty pointless. She took my temperature, changed my bandage and told me about the American Cancer Society Reach for Recovery Program, which, when I felt a little better, I did visit.

Lots of cards, flowers and candy arrived at the house. Each one was appreciated and offered a lift. This kind of experience clarifies who your friends are and the importance of family. You get to see who shows up for you and how much you are loved. That part can be very life-affirming.

The next weekend Pam came to visit me in Michigan. We went out to dinner with my nieces and while it was summer and everyone else was tan I looked corpse-like, nearly transparent. I wore a big sweater and scarf to hide the surgery and my appetite was nil. I moved like an 80-year-old woman. The surgery, pain, drain and allergic reaction pretty much wiped me out. It was all I could do to get through dinner. I say this to let you know that feeling like a truck ran you over is not unusual. The pain medicine can mask what is really going on, but don't expect to feel like doing much for a number of weeks.

Two weeks after the surgery I did go to the American Cancer Society Reach for Recovery office, over in Flint. The shock of having had a mastectomy was still fresh and I felt fragile. A woman sat with me and we talked about my experience. She was a breast cancer survivor too. She offered me a couple of comfortable bras and some stuffing for them. I had to laugh. Last time I put stuffing in a bra I think I was a 12-year-old-girl. She gave me phone numbers of women who would call me if I wanted. I said okay, sure. I left with my little package. Over the next couple of weeks I did have a couple of conversations with their volunteers.

TIP: The American Cancer Society's Reach for Recovery Program is a great resource. The staff offers counseling, information and support and will give you bras that are comfortable to wear post-surgery.

Dr. Arora, the medical oncologist in Michigan, wanted me to do chemotherapy. His reasoning was that even though the size of any one of my tumors wasn't two centimeters (the point at which they would advise chemotherapy) when you added them up it was more than two centimeters. I decided that I would wait and discuss it with my oncologist in Los Angeles as I wouldn't be undergoing the chemo here in any case. The fact that the cancer wasn't in my lymph nodes gave me a feeling I had some time plus I just was not up to it. Maybe later. It was then that I thought about all the women that don't feel they have a choice, or much time to adjust.

TIPS: If you have a mastectomy ask for help with the swelling. Take your pain medicine as directed. You don't want the pain to get ahead of you. And ask your doctor about taking a laxative or stool softener. The pain medicine shuts everything down and a stool softener may be necessary for your comfort. Be exceedingly careful with the drain. It is a two-way street for germs and infection. Keep it dry and clean. If the drain clouds up get the doctor to check it immediately. Mine got cloudy, like a milkshake, and put me back in the hospital. If you have a fever or the area gets red or warm call your doctor immediately.

Getting an infection is nothing to take lightly as it too can be life-threatening and, in many cases necessitates the removal of the expander/implant in order to cure it, which means another operation. For me it came on suddenly.

I remember specifically the days and nights three weeks after the mastectomy when the infection took over my body. While I was feeling incredible fatigue for a week the obvious symptoms came on within half an hour. It was a Sunday and I had just taken my niece to meet a friend and had driven about 40 minutes away from the house. I thought if I felt strong enough I would stop and shop for a bit, longing to get my life back to normal as soon as possible. After I dropped her off I got back into the car and instantly felt overcome with debilitating fatigue. I decided I'd better just get home. By the time I reached the house I was visibly shaking with fever. The fever was raging (104 degrees) and the chills shook my body so violently I felt like a character out of *The Exorcist*. The fever and the shaking just got worse over the next hour. Fred was home that day and he took me to the emergency room.

I have never been so sick in my life. That afternoon I was immediately put on intravenous antibiotics but not before I vomited a few times once, for the record, all over my brother's arm. I remember thinking, "Good thing he puts his hands in people's chests for a living," as he was not offended by my getting sick all over him. I felt like a dishrag. That night when the hospital finally found a room for me, I lay back in the bed, which felt like a cloud from heaven after being on an emergency gurney for five hours. I started to think that was why gurneys are so uncomfortable – to make you appreciate their less than stellar beds.

Fred looked at me with my hair plastered to my head from sweat and in an unattractive hospital gown and said, "You want anything from home? A brush?" I am sure I looked like a refugee. "No, nothing," I replied weakly. He looked at me incredulously, "Nothing?" I had come to the hospital with just the clothes on my back. This from a sister who is not inclined to "pack light" and loves to read. No, I didn't want to be burdened with any possessions. I didn't want anything to touch my skin. I didn't want to be faced with any choices. I just wanted to sleep. There was nothing of this world that would have made me feel better. It was an effort to lay my head on the pillow.

That night, once the shaking stopped, I was as close to "nothing" as I have ever been. My body and mind were depleted, reduced. What was previously strong had no strength, what was previously important had no pull over me. I was, as author Eckhart Tolle would say, "just being." Complete surrender, not out of choice but because there was no other alternative and yet, in the surrender, I finally did feel peaceful.

There was, oddly, freedom with everything stripped away. All my illusions of control were replaced with acceptance. Clearly I was not in control, this was not of my choosing...none of it. Earlier, in the chaos of being so sick, I didn't realize it was such a deconstruction process. The infection had systemically alerted all the cells in my body. I felt I wasn't hitting bottom so much as hitting essence. The truth is, I've never felt so in touch with my soul as that first night, when I was hooked up to an IV but needed and wanted nothing else. I was nearly just spirit, meditative, housed in the shell of my body, on the edge. I swear, a faint wind and I would have been gone.

TIP: Infection is a real threat and can have long-term consequences. Systemic infections can lead to loss of limb and/or life. The symptoms of fever and shakes are hard to ignore but it is best if it doesn't get to this stage. If the draining fluid isn't clear get it checked out immediately. A warm or red breast is also a sign of trouble and needs to be examined immediately.

For a long week, the heavy-duty antibiotic pumped through my system. If it didn't get the infection under control the doctors were going to have to remove the implant and start over after it healed. Thank God for the summer Olympics of 2004 – it was the only thing that kept me sane. Why can't hospitals have a better TV service and what about a Laugh Channel?

It is so obvious to me now that a healthy person is vibrating at a different frequency than an ill one. Try as you might, you have really no frame of reference for the sick. Conversely, when you are diminished from illness you look at the healthy and think, "Why are they moving so fast?" As nurses or doctors rush into a room, full of energy and good health, you feel they are more like aliens.

I remembered the previous year when my sister-in-law was dying of cancer. She looked so uncomfortable. I wanted to make it better for her but she didn't want anything. I was full of questions. Can I make you tea? Water? Do you want me to fix the pillow? Do you want to watch TV? I was floundering for ideas. She was dying. I understand that a bit better now. Now I know just being with the person can be enough. In my experience the presence of calm, healthy energy without any obvious action related to it can be comforting to the sick. Holding the space for healing is an act of grace.

TIP: If you are caretaking, sometimes just your company will be all that is needed, nothing more.

The nursing shifts changed at the hospital at 11:00 P.M. and the noise and commotion woke me nightly. I've been to Hollywood parties that were quieter. The nurses and staff need to exchange information but it is more like a celebration for the nurses who are leaving and a shot of adrenaline for the ones taking over. My room was right across from the nurses' station and the noise seemed to go on for an hour or more. This happened every night for the week I was there. Are they unaware that there are sick people who need their rest? Or don't they care? Why is there is so little consideration for someone sleeping in a modern hospital?

It appears as though a sleeping patient is seen as an inconvenience – hard to get a blood pressure reading when the patient is asleep. Why else would they wake you at 5:30 A.M. to take blood? I know the hospital is their work environment but to patients it is their temporary home. Here are my five wishes regarding nursing care – *lower your voice, wash your hands with hot water, ask permission before you touch, explain what you are going to do before you do it and let sleeping patients sleep.*

On Friday I arranged to have someone from a local salon come in and wash my hair as I couldn't do it with the IV attached and the nurses didn't offer to help. Fred came into my room at the end of the day. I asked him how his day went. He said, "Good. Did two hearts today" (he performed two coronary artery bypass operations). He asked me, "How was your day? What did you do?" Proudly I said, "I got my hair washed." I don't know who felt more accomplished.

Over the weekend I was finally discharged. The infection had been brought under control but had made the area more painful. It was still touch and go as to whether the implant would have to be removed and I would have to start over.

TIP: If you don't have family able to help you wash your hair in the hospital you can sometimes call someone from a local salon to come and do it for you. I personally think hospitals should have a salon facility so someone can get their hair washed if necessary, especially if you are there for an extended stay. It seems like basic care to me but I have found many nurses don't seem to have the time or inclination to help with personal hygiene.

PAIN MANAGEMENT

Pain is the great debilitator. It makes you slow down, sometimes to a crawl, and not just physically but mentally. Clearly, pain often leads to depression, and chronic pain

can feel intolerable at times. And it is one of the great fears, spoken and unspoken, of cancer patients – the pain associated with the disease.

The great news about modern medicine is that modalities are available to block or at least manage most physical pain. The bad news is that the people administering the drugs are often not in tune with what is actually going on with the patient and are stuck on protocols that aren't necessarily helpful. And a patient's condition is fluid, so adjustments need to be made consciously and frequently to adequately address the pain effectively while not suppressing respiratory function to a dangerous level.

Jeffrey Mogil, Ph.D., director of the Pain Genetics Laboratory at McGill University in Montreal, is studying pain and how differently the genders respond to it. His work suggests that neural pathways differ in men and women and therefore the pain drug one would create based on a particular protein would differ. He says, "Women are more sensitive to pain than men and they have a higher ability to discriminate among different pain levels." Estrogen seems to increase pain sensitivity while testosterone seems to diminish the sensitivity.

In many ways alleviating pain is not just a science but an art, and it requires finesse. Pain medications can be dangerous if mixed with other drugs so you should not be your own "prescriber." You need expert advice and counsel. A cocktail of the wrong meds can kill you. There are many tragic examples where mixing medicines, any medicines, including the over-the-counter variety, proved fatal.

So many people are on various daily drugs that any pain

medicine needs to be taken cautiously and with a doctor's prescription and supervision. And it is absolutely necessary that you be honest and forthright with your doctors about what you are taking, including anything over-the-counter or herbal. The doctor's advice and recommended protocol is based to some degree on the information which they are given. There is a public misconception that over-the-counter medicines or herbal medicines are harmless, perhaps because they are readily available or considered "natural" but all medicine has side effects and combining any medicine, over-the-counter or prescription, without a doctor's approval is dangerous. Tylenol PM and the like are easily bought but they are also powerful, and just because they can be obtained without a prescription does not make them harmless; they can be a toxic combination when mixed with other meds.

Pain management is certainly an area where you need to speak up. You are the only one who can say how the medicine is affecting you. I for one was told many times to "take two Vicodin every four hours as needed for pain." This didn't work for me. The sudden surge of that much Vicodin in my system made my skin itch at the onset and wore off too quickly so that by the end of the four hours I was in agony again. Instead, I took the pills and split them in half and took a half every hour. It was the same amount of medicine but the delivery of a constant and smaller dose worked much more effectively for me. I could only do this at home because when you are in the hospital they *make* you take the prescription medicine while they watch you. You can't arbitrarily keep the pills and take them as you wish due to prescription pain medicine controls. Of course giving you medicine *once* every four hours is more efficient for *them* so they aren't eager to change the delivery system. Again, you have to be the judge and ask for something different from your doctor if it isn't working for you. If the doctor leaves different orders then the medicine delivery will be adjusted, but without a change in the prescription the nurses have no control over altering your medication.

TIP: Drugs are available to manage most pain but they need to be administered in a way you can tolerate. What you have "onboard" – the term for how much pain medicine is in your system – needs to be regulated in an individual way. This is not one size fits all. In order to get your pain medicine protocol refined, you will need to let your doctor know it isn't working for you, otherwise you will get the standard dosage. Lack of pain control is a top complaint in hospitals but much can be done. The doctors are always balancing adequate respiratory function with pain control.

This is also true for pain medicine that doesn't agree with you. Not everyone has the same reaction to Percocet, morphine, Vicodin, and Darvon. I personally dread the feeling morphine brings. It is a powerful pain reliever and when you need it you are thankful for it, but as it collects in your system the effects can be very uncomfortable. The hand-delivery pump system (PCA or patient-controlled analgesia) is an efficient system in that it can provide a continuous small dose of medication, which you yourself can augment by pressing a button. You cannot overdose yourself since it is strictly programmed with lock-out intervals and maximum totals over time. Unfortunately the instructions you receive are not always clear.

NOTE TO DOCTORS, NURSES AND ANYONE ELSE CARETAKING:

Bedside manner starts when you walk into a patient's room. We hear about the concept when it comes to doctors but it really applies to any caretaker or for that matter *anyone* who has contact with the patient. *Are you being consciously*

responsible for the attitude and energy that you bring into the patient's room?

What seems to be required is "presence." I've experienced it myself and seen it with others. When doctors and staff are "present" to the patient, the energy in the room shifts. Patients, for lack of a better word, exhale. They feel listened to. Simple acts like eye contact and addressing the patient by name should not be minimized. Charts and hospital notes are important but distracting. Also, slow it down. Doctors are so busy with a schedule that would choke an elephant and nurses are dealing with more duties than ever, that it is hard for nurses and doctors to slow down enough to spend the time to answer questions and reassure. Third, appropriate touching to diagnose or check a wound is important but there is a caveat: ask permission first! It is hard to care for someone at arm's length however; the power of touch is just that...powerful. No touching without asking the patient if you can, and be as explicit as possible as to what you are planning on doing. Removing a drain, taking off a bandage, taking blood all become less traumatic if the patient has been told exactly what is intended and agrees to the intended action before proceeding. As a caretaker you have no right to assume the patient is ready for you to act, you must ask.

I agree with Jill Bolte Taylor, Ph.D., who writes in her book, *My Stroke of Insight*, as patients I think we want our doctors to "protect us not just probe us." She further writes, "I realized that morning that a hospital's number one responsibility should be protecting its patients' energy levels."

Doctors do not heal but rather their job is to inspire and facilitate in the healing. The healing has to come from

the patient. What I know is when you are using all your energy to heal, bad medicine and bad bedside manners act as energy drainers. Heightened anxiety in an existing tense situation only pushes up blood pressure, raises heart rate and pumps adrenaline into a body that is already challenged. Doctor-patient interaction isn't just a human issue but a medical issue. And these moments when anxiety is high correlate with pain response. If hospitals are serious about pain control, which is the number one complaint among patients in hospitals, then the issue of bedside manner should not be overlooked or underestimated and nuts and bolts training in people skills of all medical staff is essential.

TIP: Something no one warns you about but every post-mastectomy patient I have talked to experiences, and finds really uncomfortable, is what I term the "deep itch" that comes along with the healing. I believe it comes from nerve endings re-firing but when it occurs under the implant it is impossible to scratch the itch. I found ice packs help.

Once it was clear that the infection was gone and the expander could remain in, my plastic surgeon, Dr. Alghanem, would fill the expander implant with saline through the port. This once-a-week routine reminded me of when the orthodontist would tighten my braces – *oweeee!* It didn't hurt much as he filled it but would ache afterwards as the chest wall and the skin felt the need to stretch. He was pumping me up to get to the D size that would match my right side in a bra. It looked much like the scene in *Pulp Fiction* – a hypodermic needle in the chest only it was just saline delivered through a port in the implant. As he filled it weekly, I grew, and I looked more normal in clothes. Naked it was as uneven as could be – one side hard and upright, the other soft and natural. Only with a bra on did I feel balanced. I found this so disconcerting that I even slept wearing a soft fabric bra to keep my chest in place.

SALINE IMPLANTS WITH PORTS

A saline implant that is also an expander is used to expand the skin and muscle slowly, every week adding more saline though a small port that is visible but covered by skin. If you decide on saline implants they can be left in permanently. In that case, the doctor would just remove the port and you are done. A saline implant does not feel as comfortable as silicone, often creating a shape that is rounder and harder and looking more like a water balloon. A saline implant will look and feel less like your natural breast than silicone. But for some women who do not want to be concerned with any of the possible side effects of silicone, saline is a good alternative.

By the way, if you have girlfriends with saline or silicone implants purely for augmentation, you cannot compare their experience with yours. Since they did not have mastectomies there would still be breast tissue covering the implants which makes for a whole different look and feel. At the time of my mastectomy (2004) silicone was still not approved for regular use and my first plastic surgeon, Dr. Alghanem, would not consider using them at all. Silicone was always readily available for mastectomy patients in Europe but not always in the U.S. But since the saline expander can be increased in size by adding more saline through a port and the silicone is a fixed size, usually a saline expander implant is used first in mastectomy cases to create the right size pocket, and then later replaced, at the patient's option, with silicone. Of course this means an additional operation is required if you want to replace it with silicone later. New techniques have been developed since my surgery that would require only one surgery and are discussed later in this book.

In my case the drain continually irritated the area under the implant which caused it to produce excess fluid and I never got under the recommended amount. Finally a decision was made, seven weeks after the surgery, to take the drain out. I instantly felt better, my body equalizes and fifteen pounds lighter, the good news, I finally returned to Los Angeles.

NOTE: Years later, in 2008, I asked Dr. Alghanem what his concerns were with me at the time of surgery. His biggest issue was my irradiated breast tissue. Once the tissue has been exposed to radiation there is always a worry about healing, and specifically capsular contraction. In my case the irradiated breast actually healed better with less scaring, but that isn't always the case.

When I asked him if he had ever done a reconstruction and a reduction at the same time he responded in the negative. His view was that wasn't a good idea. The length of time of the surgery, the difficulty of establishing symmetry, the healing that needs to take place and the additional chance of PE (pulmonary embolism) and increased bleeding all contribute to added risk.

I asked him about his most pressing concern when counseling patients who come to him for reconstruction. He made it clear that his first priority is their safety, and that it is vital the reconstruction will not impact their cancer treatment. He also wants to evaluate their motivation for the reconstruction surgery to make certain that it is the woman's decision and she is not being coerced by others. Further, he wants to warn patients that implant surgery is a lifelong concern: the implants need to be maintained and monitored and will need to be replaced if there is leakage or after a number of years. And, that while the goal is to achieve symmetry, the implant side will not be as it was before surgery. "Even the symmetry that you

might have right after surgery is not permanent. Weight changes and aging will continue to impact long-term results."

In his practice, 10-15% of the women he counsels decide not to go ahead with the reconstruction after hearing all the issues related to the procedure. If a patient decides to go ahead with the reconstruction they will be given a multiple-page informed consent form from the American Society of Plastic Surgeons to fill out.

When I got back to Los Angeles my first appointment was with Dr. Van Scoy-Mosher, at Cedars-Sinai Medical Center in Beverly Hills, my oncologist. He examines me and we talk about chemotherapy. He does not think the benefits outweigh the risks in my case. He advises me to go on tamoxifen. His nurse checks my blood markers, which by the way have remained normal during this whole ordeal. I will have to have my blood checked every three months. I decide against the tamoxifen for now.

WHAT IS CHEMOTHERAPY?

Chemotherapy is a systemic drug treatment to kill cancer cells. If it is administered before surgery, to shrink the tumor, it is called neoadjuvant chemotherapy. When a tumor is large this is often recommended. If it is given after surgery, which is most common, it is called adjuvant chemotherapy.

The drugs that are used are called cytotoxic drugs: *cyto*, Latin for cells, and toxic. If you are already sick, why take toxic substances into your system? Because they kill rampant, errant cancer cells. In this process good cells will be killed as well, which is why you may lose your hair

and eyelashes. Chemotherapy is especially hard on fast-growing cells. Cancer cells, as well as the cells that grow your hair, are fast-growing cells. Your hair will grow back. Hopefully the cancer cells will be gone for good.

If there is lymph node involvement, chemotherapy is routinely recommended. The purpose is to kill any cancer cells that have traveled beyond the breast and the lymph nodes. These cancer cells may be microscopic in nature but there is no way of detecting where they are hiding. If there isn't lymph node involvement then other factors are weighed and the decision can be more complicated and more subjective.

A chemotherapy regimen is a cocktail of cytotoxic drugs individually designed for you and given in cycles. There is no such thing as one-size-fits-all chemotherapy. Some treatments are intravenous; some are taken by mouth. Generally chemotherapy is administered in a series of treatments over a period of weeks or months.

Chemotherapy is sometime prescribed even when there is no evidence of cancer outside the breast. This is determined often by the size of the tumor and the tumor pathology. The purpose would be to destroy any micronmetastases that may be too small to be discovered by tests that are currently available.

"Dose dense" chemotherapy is when drugs are given more frequently than the traditional cycle. For this protocol, doctors will need to evaluate your tolerance to the drugs and monitor you very carefully, watching especially that your blood count levels do not get too low.

IF CHEMOTHERAPY HAS BEEN PRESCRIBED WHAT DO YOU NEED TO DO?

Mouth Care and Oral Health

Ask your doctor about seeing a dentist before starting chemotherapy. Your mouth can be greatly affected by the chemo and knowing that your mouth and teeth are healthy prior to starting treatment is a good idea. Chemotherapy can increase decay so you want your mouth to be in optimum health. Preventionmouthrinse.com and Biotene.com are two good sources of information. Talk to your oncologist about this before you see the dentist and get a recommendation.

Organize a Schedule of Help and Support

Coordinate who will be taking you to chemotherapy, staying with you during your treatment and driving you home, and perhaps even staying overnight. Coordinate any other logistics that need to be taken care of like grocery shopping, laundry, child care or housekeeping. Stock up on dry goods such as toilet paper and light food, things like crackers and soups.

Shop

Do you think you may want a wig? If so, look into getting a wig before your hair begins to fall out. Doing this before the hair loss may make the shopping experience a bit better. You can also better match your style and color if you decide to stay with your current hairstyle. And it could be a nice time to try a different look and become a blonde or long and curly when you have always had short straight brown hair. For some, making this time

really different physically (being a blonde when you were always a redhead) makes it have bookends – a beginning and an end.

WHAT ARE THE TYPICAL SIDE EFFECTS OF CHEMOTHERAPY?

Chemotherapy is feared almost as much as the cancer. It has a notorious reputation as most everyone is aware of the effects of chemo, as it's used on all kinds of cancer, not just breast cancer. The head scarf and translucent skin are all too common a sight in America.

You may experience some or all of these side effects. All side effects and unusual responses during this time should be discussed with your physician. You are in a compromised state and how your individual body reacts to the drugs cannot be predicted. It is important not to ignore side effects and to advise your doctor exactly as to what you are experiencing. Infection is always a possibility, a dangerous one, and it is important to be monitored closely at this time.

Hair Loss

This is one side effect that saddens and terrifies women. Historically, as women, we are attached to our hair. The only good news about losing your hair is that it does grow back – unlike a breast. The bad news is that when you are already feeling your worst, you lose what has always been one of the symbolic cornerstones of your femininity. Literally, it could be bad hair days on steroids.

I know women who reject chemotherapy because they don't want to lose their hair. If chemotherapy is what is

being offered to you by knowledgeable doctors then to forego the treatment just to keep your hair isn't wise. I don't underestimate how hard this change is especially when you are already feeling under attack but the fact is, they don't have many options to offer you. They need to kill the microscopic cells that may be lurking in places that only chemotherapy can reach.

Of course there are wigs you can wear, and hats, and scarves but you know and I know it won't be the same until you get through the treatments and your hair grows back. Again we can only hope for more targeted treatments in the future so that hair loss won't be part of the side effects.

And hair loss will likely include your eyelashes and eyebrows and any other body hair you may have. As mentioned earlier, the reason is chemotherapy kills fast-growing cells and hair is made up of them – they are in the crossfire. On a positive note, some women like to use the symbolism of hair loss as an indication that the chemotherapy is indeed doing what it was intended to do – kill fast-growing cells – but the effects are not easy to live with regardless.

Many have said that a proactive approach to hair loss is best. Shaving it off before it falls out makes you feel like you have some control. Or cut it short and get used to short hair before it starts to fall out. This way you can also try out a hairstyle that could be possible once it grows back.

Weight Gain or Loss

Ask your doctor about your weight and what you might anticipate in terms of weight loss or gain. A myth about chemotherapy is that all people lose weight during chemotherapy. The truth is some people lose weight but many others gain weight during chemotherapy. The anti-nausea drugs in combination with the steroids can make weight gain a real possibility. The misconception that you always lose weight can compound potential depression if at the end of your treatment you are much heavier than you anticipated. Your first priority is getting through your treatment, no matter your weight, but having a conversation with your doctor before you start can eliminate any unnecessary surprises when it comes to weight.

Nausea and Vomiting

The chemotherapy disrupts your digestion. A common and unpleasant side effect is nausea. Anti-nausea drugs have become much more effective in recent years. Consult with your doctor as they may be able to adjust your drugs and make you more comfortable. Zofran by GlaxoSmithKline (generic ondansetron) is a popular anti-nausea medicine. Emend (aprepitant) by Merck is another one.

Tingling or Numbing of the Hands or Feet

Chemotherapy affects your nerves, which means tingling or numbing of your hands and feet is something you may experience. Neuropathy is a side effect that can outlast the treatment and linger to some degree or another so this is not a minor side effect and should be brought to the attention of your physician immediately.

Mouth Sores

Mouth sores are not to be minimized. Let your physician and dentist know that you are experiencing these symptoms as they can be painful and need attention. While it is good to drink water the chemo can leave you with a metal taste in your mouth. Slightly flavored waters, teas by Arizona or Sobe, and lightly flavored drinks may be a way to increase your liquids without drinking plain water. Sparkling water that is lemon or lime flavor is another possibility. It is important to stay hydrated.

Dry Mouth

Biotene Toothpaste for Dry Mouth, Biotene Gel for Dry Mouth, Tom's Natural products and lemon non-sugar mints have been known to be helpful.

Depression

There is an emotional component of chemotherapy and again the response can be as individual as you are. Some patients have a hard time with the drugs entering their body, fearing more damage to tissue and organs. Some patients have difficulty with the physical changes that are going on – the loss of hair and bloating due to the drugs. Others have had only a short amount of time to get their arms around the idea that they have cancer and that alone can bring on depression. Honestly, there is plenty to be depressed about and seeking professional emotional support during this time should be considered if you are feeling overwhelmed. Family and friends can of course, be helpful but sometimes their best efforts fall short.

If you don't have access to private professional help there are support groups like American Cancer Society's Reach for Recovery and the Wellness Center that can offer some relief. In many cases just talking to a survivor can be enormously

helpful. The resource guide in the back of this book offers some places where you may be able to get support.

Fatigue

You will be tired, no doubt. This is the time to do the minimum and not burden yourself with anything extra. If you can nap, nap. If you can get some help with housework and child care, get it. You will likely not have the energy to do your normal routine so just know this is no time to be Superwoman.

Dark Veins and Nails

The chemotherapy can make your veins dark. This can become more apparent as your skin may appear to be more translucent due to the drugs.

Low White Blood Cell Count

Your white blood cells ward off infection and should be monitored very carefully by your doctor. Most likely drugs will need to be administered to keep your white blood cell count high enough to enable you to continue with chemo. These may be shots that you will administer to yourself. And as a result of chemotherapy your immune system is compromised, which makes you susceptible to infection. Stay away from others who have colds or flu and wash your own hands frequently.

Possible Early Menopause

Chemotherapy can cause women to enter early menopause resulting in hot flashes and night sweats. Any concerns

about this needs to be discussed with your physician prior to beginning chemotherapy.

Loss of Fertility

Besides early menopause, chemotherapy and other hormonal treatments may cause infertility. The possibility of this happening to you should be discussed with your doctor *prior to beginning your treatment.* Doctors are generally focused on your disease and not your fertility so if this is important to you, make sure that it gets discussed openly so you know what to expect. The loss of fertility to a woman wanting to have her own biological children should not be dismissed as "irrelevant" just because there is disease. The emotional component of this side effect is underestimated and the medical community needs to be more sensitive to this issue. However saving a life always has to be the priority.

Sexual Side Effects

Lack of libido due to the emotional as well as the physical effects of chemotherapy can have an impact on sexual responsiveness. Some women during and after chemotherapy experience the physical side effect of vaginal dryness which can make intercourse painful. There are various lubricants on the market which can help to alleviate some of these physical symptoms such as Replens or Astroglide. Again, the emotional component is complicated to dissect and address. General feelings of fatigue and negative body image can certainly have a dramatic effect on one's feeling of sexuality and sexual desire.

CHEMOTHERAPY AND PORTS

If you have chemotherapy a port-a-cath, which is a type of central venous access catheter, may be recommended for you. A port is a device that is inserted into a central vein in your chest temporarily so that they can administer the chemotherapy and test your blood via a small needle which is inserted right into the port. Multiple blood draws and chemotherapy can be particularly harsh on your veins. Many patients who have received port-a-caths are relieved at not having to endure multiple and often painful procedures of having to find a vein, cannulate it and hope the flow is good enough to either draw blood or deliver medicine. The device is temporary and will be removed after your treatment is completed. Some patients have problems with the port which needs to be brought to the attention of a doctor immediately. If it has been inserted properly and is performing properly, it should *not* be painful. But a port-a-cath does need attention and maintance.

6

Reconstruction, Reconstruction, Reconstruction

Humpty Dumpty sat on a wall
Humpty Dumpty had a great fall
All the king's horses and all the king's men
Couldn't put Humpty together again

–William Wallace Denslow, *Mother Goose*

While breast reconstruction is an option post-mastectomy not every woman chooses to undergo this procedure. Some women don't want to have more surgery; it is as simple as that. Others feel as if they have gone through too much already and don't have the financial resources or the energy to pursue this alternative. Others may still be fighting the cancer. And then there are those who don't want to have a foreign body, such as a silicone or saline implant, in their bodies. Again, this is a personal choice and only you can make it. For me, getting my body back to look as good as it could be was always the plan and a priority. But as you consider this option know it is "breast reconstruction" not "re-creation" and adjust your expectations accordingly.

My experience of undergoing several operations to get an acceptable cosmetic result is, I have come to realize, not uncommon. Either due to complications or an unsatisfactory result, many women will need to endure a series of operations. Of course, if repeated operations can be avoided, so much the better.

There were many steps in my breast reconstruction. The saline implant called an expander that was first inserted could have remained in, requiring only the removal of the port attached to the implant. But I found the saline implant uncomfortable. It always felt like a water balloon on my chest. I also found the shape of it not to be as natural as I wanted so when I got back to Los Angeles I investigated getting it replaced with silicone and having the other side reduced so that I had a more symmetrical look.

TIP: If you decide to have saline implants rather than silicone, the expander can become the final implant. Silicone implants generally cannot be inserted until the area has been previously expanded because they only come in fixed sizes. So be aware, if you choose silicone implants, it generally means a two-operation process. Note: Since the time of my surgery a new procedure with an Alloderm® matrix has been devised which can reduce the number of surgeries even if a silicone implant is used. And at the time of my surgery the stem cell procedure was also not available.

I consulted with a plastic surgeon I knew who did not do breast reconstructions, not all plastic surgeons do, and he recommended his partner. Together they met with me to discuss what they could do for me. I asked them for photos but the doctors told me, "Everyone is so different. Looking at another patient's experience isn't comparable when it comes to reconstruction." I know now that is not a good answer and I should have insisted on looking at photos or meeting with their patients. Upon agreeing to have Dr. X, (not his real name), do the surgery, his administrator told me it would cost me $5,000 out-of-pocket in addition to whatever the insurance company paid him for replacing the implant and reducing the other side.

TIP: Not all plastic surgeons perform breast reconstruction. At the very least, ask to look at photos of previous breast work (including reconstruction photos) and if they don't want to share them my suggestion is to go elsewhere. Of course, keep in mind that no one is going to show you photos of the surgeries that didn't work out. Talking to their prior patients is another good way to vet the doctor. Also valuable are recommendations from physicians you trust who are familiar with another doctor's work. Still, there are no guarantees, even after following these steps, that you will have an acceptable outcome.

TIP: Check the credentials of the surgeon. He or she should be state-licensed and "board certified," which means the doctor holds a state license to practice and has passed national examinations in that particular field. Again this does not guarantee you will be satisfied with his or her work but it does imply a certain amount of expertise.

December 7, 2004. It was a rainy day in Los Angeles. I was just a couple of days away from having the expander, which was filled with saline, taken out, and a silicone implant put in and my other breast reduced and lifted in the hopes of getting some symmetry back. I need to remember to bring my insurance card, get the house cleaned so it is nice when I get back, and shop for food I want here.

This decision to have the expander replaced with silicone turned out to be much more complicated and costly than I had first imagined. But without knowing the future you do the best you can.

TIP: Got milk? Make certain you have the essentials ready before you come home from the hospital. Light food (applesauce, cottage cheese, fruit, crackers, canned soups are all good) and something you like to drink, plenty of water at your bedside, clean towels, toilet paper, re-useable ice packs and tissues. Change the sheets before you go to the hospital so they are fresh when you come home. Have something to wear that is comfortable in bed, pillows that are firm so you can prop yourself up if necessary, cell phone and charger and telephone numbers that you might want, maybe a good book or magazines to read and buy some fresh flowers if that pleases you. If you like music set something up in your bedroom that would be soothing or have your iPod handy. If you like funny movies this would be the time to watch some of your favorites. And no cleaning the house or straining yourself: the pain killers can make you feel pain-free once they kick in but your body isn't ready for that kind of movement. Take it easy.

That afternoon I had drinks with an old college sweetheart who happened to be in town. There is nothing like an old flame to bring you back to the time when your body looked and moved like a dancer's. Oddly enough he told me his wife also had breast cancer, a very aggressive form, and she had been able to survive.

December 10, 2004. I had reconstructive surgery to replace the saline expander with the silicone implant.

December 12, 2004. I am so upset over the surgery. For some reason the whole cleavage line is wrong. It looks to me as if he didn't use the proper size implant, which really makes me furious. He reduced the right side and while it looks terrible at the moment at least I can imagine it looking okay once the scars fade. The implant side looks terrible – like a big blob on my chest that has no definition, it is too small, and the space between my breasts is wrong. I'll have to have more surgery.

TIP: When you meet with the plastic surgeon days before your scheduled surgery have him or her draw on you *exactly* what he plans to do. Yes, you will be marked up but at least you will know what to expect. And have them show you the exact size implant they will be using.

December 2004. My follow-up appointment with the plastic surgeon, Dr. X, was disappointing. He saw only his perspective. I talked only about mine – which he minimized and ignored. When he said, "Wait, let it heal," I interpreted it as, "Wait…maybe you'll get used to the result I gave you." He knew I didn't want to go through more surgery. I think he was counting on "surgery fatigue" and the possibility I would just accept the results. From my view the cleavage line was wrong. The implant was completely falling off my chest. The pocket was too big and the implant too small and unanchored. It was hard enough to accept the change that my body had gone through but I wanted an acceptable result. I admit I wanted it as good as it could be. I certainly was not going to have it falling off my chest and under my arm. I knew it wasn't going to be "normal" but this was unacceptable.

Oddly, he seemed pleased with himself and his work. It was as if his demeanor was a defense mechanism. If the result could have been better he would have been more apologetic, right? Staring at me he then says, "You must have had great breasts… the kind men stop their car for." I don't know if this was meant to embarrass me or flatter me. I couldn't believe a doctor just said that to me, "Yeah, all the more reason to get this right." I should have added "you jerk." And then I should have walked out. My Ivy League-trained L.A. plastic surgeon then said, "They are never going to be perfect." Yeah, I understand they are never going to be perfect…no kidding. Who the hell do these guys think they are talking to? I left the appointment once again not clear on what to do next.

TIP: While it is true you are picking a plastic surgeon for how they make you look not how they make you feel, if you don't have a good rapport with your doctor (any of your doctors for that matter) you will likely be frustrated. Stay focused on what the doctor is there to do for you but don't ignore an obvious disconnect. It can be hard to walk away once you have started "down the surgery road" with a doctor, financially and emotionally. But buyer beware, there is a certain amount of "selling" that is going on in these appointments and while that sounds inappropriate, to forget that medicine is also a business is naïve and not in your best interest.

2005

January 13, 2005. Due to the terrible surgery outcome I would certainly need more reconstruction and at my second meeting with the surgeon I think he agreed (although I am not absolutely clear about that, man these guys are good at ambiguity) to replace the implant. Does that mean I pay for it? I don't know. I was so tired of going under and I was not eager to have another operation but was sure I will feel up to it soon. I hated his attitude but I already paid him for this so to hire someone else meant I'd have to pay again for the same procedure as the insurance won't cover it.

In the meantime, an area next to the reduction site on my right breast was feeling hard and I planned to get that checked the following week even though the pathology report that was done at the time of the reduction came back fine. I didn't trust it. I will have Dr. Steiner put a needle in it and draw out some cells (FNA) and see what comes up. This is part of the disease…to stay vigilant.

TIP: While it is good to have options for treatment it is also difficult to know what is the right course for you. What I do know is that with every surgery there are pros and cons.

Don't be surprised if you are confused and uncertain. I haven't met anyone who has been through this who wasn't at some point.

I had a date that night with someone I didn't know well. So as I am trying to decide what to wear my mind went to the subject…do I tell, when do I tell, it isn't any of his business right? God I hope I don't want to sleep with him soon because then I will have to tell. Right? Or do I keep a bra on and the lights off. Will he care? Of course he'll care. Will any man care? Will any man care enough for me that he won't care about the breast cancer? As if I didn't have enough to think about. Should I cancel the date? If they fall in love with me before I tell them, is that dishonest? Smart? Good timing? Dumb? I mean, after all, it isn't insignificant? I don't know. Well, I had better get dressed.

I had an appointment with Dr. Van Scoy-Mosher, the medical oncologist, scheduled for the next day to get my blood drawn.

March 7, 2005. I went to see both Dr. X and Dr. Van Scoy-Mosher, my oncologist. The appointment with the plastic surgeon was as expected. He took no responsibility for the fact that it was not right and told me, "how much of an improvement it had been (over the expander)" and that "all women that come in here want a normal breast, and that just isn't going to happen." The last comment I find particularly insulting. Why are doctors like this in women's health? I needed to find someone else to fix this.

Dr. Van Scoy-Mosher, my oncologist at Cedars-Sinai, I find to be an exception to this kind of callousness and I have found him compassionate. My appointment was for "routine" blood work. As soon as I entered his waiting room at Cedars-Sinai Medical Center it is clear there is nothing routine about this. I am still so accustomed to being healthy all my life I felt as though I don't fit in.

It all reminds me of a joke Norman Lear told me once about the surprise of getting older. When he was 60 years old he came home one day and heard his friends gathered in the living room. As he walked into the room he saw a bunch of "old" people. His first reaction was, "What are all my parents' friends doing in my living room?" So yes, my first reaction is always, "What am I doing with all these sick people?"

Dr. Van Scoy-Mosher examined me. He told me once again that I should go on tamoxifen if only to reduce my chances of getting cancer in the other breast. I told him I would think about it.

His nurse took more of my blood. It had been recommended that my blood be tested every three months. She told me it "looked good." I asked her to explain the numbers to me. I always wanted to know what made it 'good.' So-called tumor markers are low and usually mean there is no cancer. High or elevated tumor markers would indicate the disease has recurred somewhere in the body. Tumor markers are not always helpful in the initial diagnosis of a cancer, because they are frequently normal; but once the cancer has been treated they are used as a tool to detect if the cancer has erupted again and/or spread. However just because your markers are normal does not mean you don't have cancer. It just means it hasn't spread to the degree that it can be picked up in your blood. My markers were normal throughout this whole ordeal. Blood work when your numbers were never high even though you had cancer hopefully tells you more of the same – you get to keep on living with just the fear but not the cancer.

Remember my date? Well things have progressed. So now I may have to take my clothes off. You've got to be kidding!

In 2004 while I went through the four surgeries including the mastectomy I was no longer in a relationship. My long-time boyfriend and I had broken up in October of '03 and while I dated there was no one in the "partner" department whom I could count on during that year. In some ways of course this made the experience incredible lonely and depressing but in other ways it freed me to just take care of my emotional needs and not worry about how someone else was coping. If I wanted to go to bed in the least sexy but coziest nightgown I could find I wasn't letting anyone else down, I didn't have to engage sexually, I didn't have to make sure he wasn't being inconvenienced by my illness and I didn't have to worry about him. Of course, I also had to do it – the healing – without someone rubbing my back, bringing me flowers, calling me just to see how I was doing, making fun of the hospital with me (how does someone ever get better here?) or bringing me popsicles and ice packs.

I didn't have children to deal with either, a subject I am going to leave for another person to discuss because I have no reference for how that impacts everything. I just had me and my wonderful friends, family and my dog but when you are 48 and not involved with anyone and going through something like this no matter how much your friends and family want to be there for you, lacking a partner can make you feel more isolated than you can imagine, especially if you are used to having one. Time and possessions change their meaning and their relationship to you when your body is fighting for its very survival. It is as though you are "divorcing" your previous life and in many ways it mirrors a marital divorce. "Recovery" was my partner. I spent a lot of time alone with the recovery.

All this alone time helped get me back to my life now. To what is supposed to be normal. The thought of another man entering my life filled me with trepidation. How would I explain this and how would he react? I knew before I even put myself out there in the dating world that I would have to be really centered about this. Like any physical change that was not of your own making a level of acceptance is necessary. Clearly, if a man didn't have the ability to accept this he would not be right for me and even if he did accept it he still might not be right for me but acceptance would be essential. I thought a lot about how I would feel if I were a man or how I would feel about anything physically challenging that a man now brought to the table.

Ironically, many years ago I did have a relationship with a man who had testicular cancer and I do remember how hesitant he was about telling me. As though having only one testicle was going to "turn me off." The only part that concerned me was that I was getting involved with someone that had had cancer. What if he gets it again? What if I am in love with him and he dies? But a testicle is not a breast and men are not women.

I have to say the man I dated next was pretty wonderful about the news. When it was clear the relationship was getting physical and that nakedness may come into the equation I knew I had some explaining to do.

Fully clothed I said, "Hey, I need to tell you something." His first reaction was "Uh-oh. Don't tell me you're involved with someone else?" "No, no one else." I had to smile. I wish that was it. "Well, what then?" he asked. Deep breath, "I've had breast cancer. I had to have a mastectomy last year." He looked at me, his arms were around me and he said, with an English accent I might add, "It doesn't matter a bit to me. I mean, I'm sorry you had to go through that but it doesn't matter to me about your breast." The total acceptance brought relief. It certainly made me want to love him. It didn't work out that way. I didn't fall in love with him in spite of his acceptance but he did make me realize it was going to be okay. That life, one including sex and partnership, was possible.

April 2005. There was another lump I was concerned about on my right breast. It was a nodule by the scar of the reduction. It was hard like a pea and I just didn't like it. I didn't have any of the "feelings of activity" that I had with the other breast, thank goodness, but given my history it made me wonder. I made an appointment to see Dr. Steiner.

TIP: Know what is or feels new or different about your body and what has always been there. And when there is a change get it checked out. Be aware of the uniqueness

of your own body. You have been living in this body and know its idiosyncrasies. Doctors can be wonderful in their ability to diagnose a problem but they are not know-it-alls – far from it.

At the appointment Dr. Steiner looked at my breasts and frankly said, "They aren't pretty, are they?" as if I needed confirmation. Shaking my head I agreed, "I know, I need to get them fixed." Sounds like I am talking about my car. He put a needle in the lump. The results of that turned out to be fine but he thought I should have a more in-depth ultrasound done. I made an appointment at the Mark Taper's Foundation Imaging Center at Cedars-Sinai Medical Center.

TIP: Check if you have reached your insurance maximum amount for the year – the threshold at which the insurer starts to pay 100% for the balance of the year. Insurance companies do not send you a notice when you reach it (they should of course) and the hospitals have this information as well as the insurance company. It may impact your decisions regarding the timing of your treatment and any other medical needs you have to take care of prior to the start of a new year. If you have treatment in one "insurance year" you will incur less of out of pocket expense.

I called the facility the day before to get a price on the ultrasound. I was still not up to my maximum "out of pocket" for the year, which was $5,000 meaning I would have had to pay 30% of the costs. The Imaging Center never called me back so I when I arrive at the Mark Taper building for my appointment I asked the staff how much it was going to cost. They looked at me strangely, as though they had never heard the question before, and then took me to a cubicle and opened a huge book and looked up the code. Every device and procedure has a billing code. For an ultrasound on one breast they would charge my insurance $990.00. I thought the amount outrageous and left without letting them do it.

Hospital pricing is the dirty big secret of the medical community. Why is it that hospitals are the only places on earth where you don't know what something costs before you buy it?

I can't tell you how many doctors have asked me, "You have insurance don't you?" As if that is all you need. That is no longer the case if you have a serious illness. The insurance coverage can leave you with a huge bill – your co-pay – because the cost they are quoting to the insurance company is inflated.

Hospitals make no effort to tell you how much something is going to cost upfront because they know that might discourage you from not only having the procedure but, more importantly to them, having the procedure at their facility. Yet, when the bill comes, and it is always more than you expected, they have no trouble harassing you for payment.

This system is a relic of simpler times. Until consumers insist and Congress passes laws to make hospitals comply, they will continue to hide their fees. This works to their advantage because you as the consumer do not question the outrageous amounts hospitals are charging because many of us rely on "magical thinking" and believe it will all be taken care of by insurance. As a matter of fact, often you have no idea what the hospital is charging. It is all smoke and mirrors until, of course, you receive a bill from the hospital two to six months later with the shock of your life. Then, if you can decipher the complicated bills, it becomes a bit clearer. But more often than not they send you a statement with an amount without the documentation to back it up.

Hospitals charge mind-popping amounts to both the insurance company and the individual without insurance. Your insurance carrier, because they contract with the hospitals, gets a discount and then pays "customary costs" but you are still stuck with a balance (your co-pay) often far in excess of what you thought the test was going to cost. And if by chance you are not in a financial position to pay this amount, hospitals have become increasingly aggressive in their efforts to collect. They will harass you day and night, garnish your wages, send you threatening letters, ruin your credit standing and generally make your life miserable. I had one hospital in Santa Monica actually say to me, "It is our policy to call the patient every week about an outstanding bill."

TIP: Before you have any procedure at a hospital or with a doctor try to determine what the actual cost will be. You may need "authorization" from your insurance company before it will agree to pay for the test or an overnight stay at a hospital. Talk to someone at the hospital financial office before you start your treatment. That person is more likely to negotiate with you *before* you have the service. Ask them what the "cash price" is and negotiate from there. And if you end up with a bill you cannot pay outright, call the hospital and ask to be put on a payment plan of a fixed amount every month.

Why isn't there an obvious medical services price list? When you make an appointment the cost of something rarely comes up if you have insurance. Routinely in hospitals as you check in you are given a piece of paper to sign accepting responsibility without any understanding of the cost, and hospitals and many doctors feel no obligation to disclose it to you. I wouldn't go to a restaurant where the menu was without prices. Let's put it this way, if I went shopping at Neiman Marcus and there were no prices on anything I think I would be far more tempted to buy their shoes, which sometimes cost as much as a refrigerator. Giving people a chance to know what something costs and allowing for a competitive decision would go a long way to fixing the system. It would create real market competition. "Health care" is also "health business" and to think otherwise is naïve. One of the first steps toward reform in my mind is to *post the costs*, at least for the standard tests and procedures.

TIP: When you are contemplating surgery make sure you get a financial quote from the anesthesiologist too. They are part of the surgery team but this specialist often bills independently from the surgeon. And also check if the anesthesiologist is in your insurance system. If you don't have insurance negotiate the fee with them upfront.

April 18, 2005. I made another appointment with a different imaging place – Beverly Hills Tower Imaging. I also asked them to call me with a price. In the four days before the scheduled ultrasound I never receive a call.

April 22, 2005. I went to Tower Imaging in Beverly Hills to get an ultrasound of my right breast. When I got there the waiting room was filled with women with anxious looks on their faces. I find even if women are in for a regular mammogram the fear of breast cancer is enough to make that furrowed line between your eyes more pronounced. Could it be the use of Botox is in direct proportion to the level of awareness of breast cancer? With 200,000 women in America diagnosed with breast cancer this year and over 40,000 deaths due to the disease the numbers are enough to turn any woman in a waiting room into a shallow breather.

On a cost mission, I asked again what Tower Imaging would charge my insurance company. I was clearly speaking with the woman who ran the office. She told me to hold on as if I was the first person who had ever asked and then looked at a small piece of paper with some prices on it. I asked her if I could have a copy of what they charge. "No, I can't give you this but I can write down what we charge." Why isn't it posted, disseminated, disclosed what they charge? Why is it a secret? When I did get the price it was one-forth of what Cedars was charging but why isn't it obvious? And why don't more people care *why* it isn't obvious?

According to the technician the ultrasound showed that that nodule was liquid and therefore not a problem. Still I wasn't completely convinced it's benign but I accepted the news.

TIP: No need to fear an ultrasound. It is non-invasive and an excellent complementary test that can usually tell if a growth is solid (tumor) or fluid (cyst). A solid mass in and of itself does not mean cancer, it just means another test may be necessary.

May 5, 2005. I feel under pressure to get this implant fixed properly as it is still unacceptable and falling off my chest but am nervous about making it even worse. At the moment I am not in pain and I don't want to be. I have another appointment with Dr. X, the plastic surgeon, thinking that I am going to make a clear decision; and sure enough once again, by the time I am ready to leave, I am just as confused as before. I don't trust him to fix it properly. He is telling me how he is going to have to make the pocket smaller and how I am not going to like how it will feel under my arm, already warning me that the outcome will be less than satisfactory. Clearly I have to research other alternatives.

I've read a lot of books lately that recognize the overwhelming nature of the "cancer experience" but emphasizing how it can result in something positive. However, the notion that it is so transformative you have to make the experience into something wonderful just adds to the pressure. That is not to say you can't have redeeming experiences along the way of this horrible journey but it is and remains horrible. Don't let anyone fool you. Maybe if you lack love in your life, you might welcome the newfound attention cancer can bring; but if you have a life and family and friends who love you, they loved you well before you had cancer. Cancer just takes the time, resources and the energy that you could have put to better use elsewhere.

This is not to say that a positive attitude isn't important but feeling as though you have to turn this into something positive and if you don't somehow you have failed the "cancer gods" is nonsense. Cancer changes you but to some degree you have no control over how it changes you. As Geralyn Lucas writes in *Why I Wore Lipstick to my Mastectomy,* you may or may not find your "inner cleavage" – a power source you didn't know you had. Or, you may be too damn tired. To the extent you do try to steer it in a positive direction, it may help your general well-being. But don't feel like you are a failure if you haven't transformed this into the best thing since on-line shopping.

I have also heard countless times in the media and elsewhere how you "have to have a good attitude." I know plenty of women with great attitudes – they still have cancer. Feel the way you feel, do what you need to do and don't let anyone tell you to have a "good attitude." Have "your attitude," one that hopefully comes from strength. Remember, everyone copes in her own individual way.

What I do think often happens is that the sudden overwhelming vulnerability you can feel makes you more open to connection. Brene Brown, a sociologist, talks about living "whole-heartedly." In her view "the way to live is to live with vulnerability." Cancer forces you to live with uncertainty, and to the degree that you accept it, is to be free. To live and love with respect but not waiting or worried about the reaction but to live in action not reaction and to understand the response is none of your business.

LINDA

I was in Malibu visiting one of my friends last week. The sky was blue, the ocean crashed on the rocks, the house was stunning. It was a perfect afternoon. "Linda" (not her real name) a beautiful woman and well-known actor, was there as well. I had spent some time with her over the years but at that point she was more of an acquaintance than a friend.

As the three of us chatted and lounged on the living room couches, Linda asked me what I had been up to. I told her last year was a wash due to my health. She asked if I was okay and I told her that yes, I was feeling better but I had had breast cancer surgery last year and the whole experience was consuming. Her next question sort of surprised me but she asked it like a veteran of the cancer wars, "Did you have to have a mastectomy?" I knew immediately she too had been through it. "Yes, I did." She continued, "Yeah me too, five years ago." I am sure my friend couldn't believe what she was hearing. Linda, whom she had known for years, had kept this from her. I could imagine her thinking, "*Not another one... she's like Susan. I can't believe women go through this and don't have the need to share it with everyone, what's with them?*"

A year later I saw Linda again. We were attending a party at the same house and as she walked directly toward me I felt there was something she needed to talk about. Sure enough, when she sat down, the horrible story she relayed deeply saddened me.

A year before, right around the time of our first conversation, she had had a lump removed which turned out to be fine. What they didn't mention at the time was that two enlarged lymph nodes were noted on the other side. It was clearly stated on the radiology report but she had never seen it or read it herself, instead relying upon her doctor to review it. Recently she had had a routine chest X-ray and they noticed again the enlarged lymph nodes except now there were even more of them. The nurse asked her why she hadn't come in sooner. Why hadn't she done anything about the 2 enlarged nodes they found earlier?

Incredulous, she went back and asked her original doctor for a copy of the radiology report. And right there in black and white the two enlarged lymph nodes were described. She immediately had surgery and an axillary node dissection. The surgeon removed all her lymph nodes on that side, 14 of which were positive for cancer. One week she thinks she's fine and the next week she has 14 nodes that are malignant. Please note: one, she never felt physically ill prior to the diagnosis and two, we are talking about some of the best doctors and hospitals in the country.

TIP: Clearly, everyone needs to read her own reports. Obvious and tragic mistakes happen.

TIP: Breast cancer generally doesn't make you feel bad physically, even if it is in your lymph system. Linda's experience is a prime example. You can absolutely have breast cancer and be asymptomatic, which is why early detection is so important.

That day, as we talked again with the ocean in the background, I saw the distress on her face. She had a five-year-old son, a horrific divorce to deal with and cancer that had spread to 14 of her lymph nodes. If she had wanted to throw the furniture off the balcony with rage it would have been understandable. Instead she sat there calmly asking me about my doctors, who I went to, who was good, what I thought.

Our friendship developed over breast cancer. We talked and met for lunch a few times as she navigated her treatment options and where to go for chemo. Luckily during this time she fell in love with a wonderful man. She finally had someone to lean on. He was the future. They made plans. They were building a life that acknowledged cancer's existence but not its virulent nature and truth – that it wants to kill you. No, when she spoke of her friend, lightness was all that was present. That love affair, her work, her brother, her friends and her little boy sustained her.

Linda was wise in that she knew that she would need help. I had offered to take her to chemo, so one day in October we went to the facility at Saint John's Health Center in Santa Monica for her fourth chemo session. They put us in a corner room with a huge view of the city. By now she knew what to expect and settled in the chair, graciously greeting all the nursing staff. Another close friend of Linda's arrived to support her. She was also a well-known actress, petite with a knockout face and a caring personality but clearly no push over. She too was a survivor. Without equivocation, this is a disease beauty does not insulate you from. Another one of Linda's tennis friends arrived and the four of us chatted and swapped stories while Linda got her chemo. We all winced as the cherry red liquid found its way into her system. And if talk could cure her we did our best that afternoon.

Women relate like fish swim. Her visitors were complete strangers to one another and yet, in the midst of someone else's suffering, we shared to entertain, distract and empathize. We could have been in a cave, in a teepee, in a modern hospital...it didn't matter. We women know how to do this by instinct. Linda's body needed healing, her spirit support, we were circling the wagons. We talked about ourselves just enough to show that we have a common experience, so Linda wouldn't feel alone and to help pass the time. We shared our experiences and our disappointments – health, men, children, our bodies...no topic taboo. Linda's vulnerability and the intimate nature of the circumstances gave us license to process our own thoughts, our own fears. We were her witnesses. It was the friendship of women being offered up as salve to the wound.

TIP: Ask for a copy of and read your own medical reports -whether lab, pathology or radiology reports, ask for and read them all! Do *not* rely just on a doctor telling you it is okay. Have them explained to you. You may not understand all of it but it forces both you and your physician to carefully go over the reports and pay attention, thereby reducing the chances of something being missed. Put copies of all reports in your health notebook for future reference. Also make sure they fax your reports to your G.P. or primary

care physician. He or she should be made aware of all your tests and results. The more people on your team who read the reports the less chance of something obvious being overlooked. You may be on medication or receive treatment for something unrelated but both could be impacted by your results or side effects. And doctors should support this kind of patient involvement as the cost of such a mistake – from malpractice to the emotional burden of making an error – is a heavy one.

In Atul Gawande's book *Better,* he writes about the 1980s case *Franklin vs. Massachusetts General Hospital* which epitomizes the devastation this simple mistake of not reading your reports can cause. Peter Franklin was discovered to have a huge tumor and Hodgkin's lymphoma. What was remarkable about this situation is that he had had his wisdom teeth removed under general anesthesia four years' prior and had had a pre-operative chest X-ray at the time at the same hospital. The X-ray indicated an abnormality and the report clearly stated, "Further evaluation of this is recommended," but the oral surgeon and surgical resident had both missed it. Instead the tumor grew untreated for four years. The additional sad irony was Peter Franklin's father was a doctor at Mass General but he too had never seen the X-ray or the report.

TIP: These records and reports do not belong to the hospital or the doctors. They are *your* reports and you are entitled to have copies of them. It is critically important to not just get a copy of any written report of a test or study; these days it is easy to obtain a CD with the actual images of the X-rays, ultrasound, CT scan, MRI, etc.

August 2005. So my campaign for truth and disclosure in hospital billing continues and heats up. I received an outrageous bill from Cedars-Sinai Medical Center for a FNA (Fine Needle Aspiration). They charged me $3,000 to put a needle in my breast and determine if any cells were abnormal. This happened in my doctor's office. He used an ultrasound machine for about 1 minute while he took the sample. They charged me for an "operating room" and $900 for the minute (literally) ultrasound and various other mind-boggling charges. The final bill to me after insurance (which paid them $1,000 for this) was $500.

I told the billing office I would not be paying it and wrote a forceful letter saying I would picket them unless they revised the bill. I am sure they will capitulate as I am certain they don't want me on the street with placards that say "Cedars Overcharges Cancer Patients." I am also sure I am not the only one where mistakes have been made. It isn't just my bill. And I know what hospitals are like if you don't pay the bill – relentless. My physician, Dr. Steiner, called me and said my letter did draw the attention of the administration and that I was "right" on this matter. That I should "give him a few days to work it out." I am tempted to have placards made and delivered to their offices to let them know I am really serious. I know Dr. Steiner knows, because he knows me, but the others don't know the fire I have for this cause. The vision of them harassing a woman still in a chemo haze over her bill (especially a mistaken one) gets me steamed.

August 13, 2005. Well, chalk up another disappointing medical experience. After waiting well over an hour beyond my appointment time to see Beverly Hills plastic surgeon Dr. K, (not his real name) I walked out. The excuse was he was running late but I think it was just business as usual. As I was waiting in the garage for my car, my cell phone rang with the office receptionist. "Susan, what happened?" she asked. She deserves the truth, right? Angry, I let her have it. "I waited over an hour for him." "Yes, he's running late," the canned excuse. "What? Does he think only his time is valuable? This is ridiculous." She starts to defend him and I cut her off. "Look, I'm looking for someone I can trust. I can't even trust him to show up for the appointment I had." She dutifully responds, "Oh, you can *trust* him." The weight of the word hung in the air. "Oh really. Well, he hasn't proven that to me. I should bill you for my time – two hours completely wasted."

My frustration over the whole experience has made me spring-loaded. What gets me really upset is I wasn't there for a nose job or Botox. I was there to get a botched breast cancer reconstruction fixed. There is a difference but that difference is apparently lost on many doctors. If I was an hour late for a real estate appointment do you think my client would wait or not expect an apology from me? It is 8:00 P.M. and he hasn't called to apologize – not that I expected him to. Like I said, business as usual.

I just finished reading a *Vanity Fair* article by Marjorie Williams detailing her battle with liver cancer. Marjorie left a husband and two kids in this world – a lot to leave. She said, "I think cancer brings to most people a new freedom to act on the understanding that their time is important." Ironic that I read this article after wasting over an hour waiting in a doctor's office waiting room. Yes, Dr. K, my time is important and if you are going to treat cancer patients you need to understand that we define it differently than most people. Not that our time is more valuable (although some would argue the point) but that our awareness of our time is more acute and therefore, we are more accountable to it. I sent Dr. K a letter outlining my disappointment and a copy of the article. I never heard another word from his office.

September 28, 2005. Last night, before bed, I realized that the diagnosis of cancer is like having a bomb in your chest without a clue as to when it will detonate. The implant, the unnatural mass that is sitting on my heart, is a constant reminder of this threat. Every twinge and slight pain gets you wondering. A headache is no longer just a headache. Is this it? Is this the moment it will all start again? What is the tipping point? What would knock the balance to trigger it...bad nutrition, stress, hormones, other medicine, aging, the silicone leaking, fear, mental attitude or none of the above? The fact is they, the experts, don't really know and you as the patient don't know either. Everyone is in the dark with the sound of the ticking. You don't want to give in to the fear but you don't want to ignore any signs either. A tightrope to be sure.

TIP: Be aware that there is an increased risk of capsular contracture if the breast has been irradiated. Capsular contracture is when the breast implant is surrounded by hardening scar tissue and "contracts" to an immovable spot on your chest. It can be painful. I did not experience this but it is something that can develop and something that you should discuss with your plastic surgeon if you are having reconstruction post-radiation or if you know you will need radiation after your reconstruction.

November 20, 2005. I found a female plastic surgeon, Dr. Barbara Hayden, who at least understood what the problems with my chest were and are. I feel heard and that was worth the $350 consultation fee. She suggested we reduce the "good" side, move the nipple and fix both folds (the place where the breast meets the chest wall so that it doesn't sink to my waist) and raise the implant side and anchor it so it doesn't move across my chest and under my arm. Finally, a voice of validation that this needs major redoing. The bad news is that her fee for this and for adding a nipple will be $17,000 and insurance will not be covering it. My insurer will pay only for "reasonable and customary" costs (its way of getting out of covering it). Regardless of insurance issues I will get newly positioned breasts (ones that actually sit on my chest) for 2006.

As I was waiting for her in the reception area there was a photograph of a woman, topless, walking on a rocky beach on the table. The inscription said, "Thanks, Dr. Hayden. We did it." I asked Dr. Hayden about the photograph. She said it was one of her post-op patients who had said, during the initial consultation, that she would deem the reconstruction a success if she could walk topless on the beach in the South of France and not feel self-conscious. It was a photo of her patient doing just that.

I wrote a letter to my previous plastic surgeon, Dr. X, telling him that I needed to have this redone and wanted my money refunded. That I didn't want to sue him but I thought it was fair that he return the cash that I paid him ($5,000 which was on top of the insurance payment) since it was such a disaster. He wrote me back that I had an "excellent" result and that he would not be refunding me any money. Pretty amazing that I needed that much correction for an "excellent" result. I didn't have the energy to fight him. You wonder how he sleeps at night.

The other turn of events is that Cedars-Sinai Medical Center, after many letters from me, finally called to discuss my bill. During this whole time the people in the billing department were sending me monthly demands to be paid and harassing me with phone calls. Can't wait to hear their explanation as to why they charged me for an "operating room" when the procedure was done in the doctor's office.

2006

March-April 2006. Cedars-Sinai Medical Center finally admits that they incorrectly billed me and decide to accept in full what the insurance already paid. It has taken 9 months, a series of letters written by me to get this bill – their mistake – resolved.

April 4, 2006. I went to another surgeon on Monday because of a lump on my right side which was suspicious on the ultrasound. Would it have been suspicious if I hadn't pointed it out? I have little faith in the "experts" "discovering" anything. Anyway, it has been decided, due to borders that look irregular (benign cysts have smooth borders) that it should come out before the reconstruction. As Dr. Hayden said, "I could take it out but I don't want to get in there and have to wait for a pathology report and if it is a problem have to change focus. I'd rather make sure it is nothing and be able to concentrate on 'pretty' during the reconstruction." I agreed. I didn't "feel" like anything was wrong and while I don't dismiss that personal assessment, I can't count on it either.

April 28, 2006. I go to the hospital in Santa Monica and have the suspicious lump taken out. They have trouble again with the IV. I have a new oncology surgeon, Dr. Maggie DiNome. She takes my Blue Cross insurance. She is smart and efficient and I see her for two minutes before I go under. Next thing I know she comes to me in the recovery area. "Good news," she says, "It looks like a former biopsy site and it looks normal." That Wednesday she calls and confirms that indeed there are no abnormal cells. The reconstruction can go ahead as planned.

May 8, 2006. So it is time for the reconstruction of the reconstruction of the reconstruction to take place. Hopefully the third time is a charm. The implant is rolling around my chest and under my arm and sinking to my waist. Nothing is anchoring it. I have a 9:30A.M. surgery in Santa Monica. This is the place where the stars have their babies. We are talking high-end health care here: America's best.

Dr. Hayden comes in, measures me with a tape measure and marks me with a hospital Sharpie. I look like a Picasso painting – all lines and circles. She knows it is going to be quite an art project to get it right. She explains that she will be putting in a new 500cc Mentor silicone implant in my chest. She tells me about lymphedema and "how important it is to elevate my left arm. If it occurs the tissue is damaged and near impossible to treat." She leaves.

I don't remember anything else until I wake up in the recovery room. It was an eight hour surgery. She had to replace the implant, remove the scar tissue, completely reconstruct a ledge for the implant to sit on and raise the other side, move the nipple and give the fold on the right side a new anchor. I was completely rebuilt from the inside out.

After the eight hour surgery I woke up in the recovery room and was in a complete panic. I looked down at my left arm and it was twice the size of normal and in it was an IV hook-up. This is the arm that I had been guarding like a bulldog and was advised by doctors for years not to even have a blood pressure cuff on that side for fear of lymphedema, and the arm Dr. Hayden had warned me, just before surgery, to treat with kid gloves. I also had another IV in my right arm and an IV in my neck which, in all the other surgeries, I had never had before. I was facing the wall, flat on my back and when I asked to see the doctor the nurses said they couldn't find her and that there were "no orders." The nurses didn't give me eye contact and hardly spoke English. They basically ignored me. I felt like a patient in a mental hospital. Meanwhile, there were men in there cleaning, I heard them dumping garbage, sweeping the floor and talking about Vietnam but they wouldn't allow my friends to come see me.

I lay there for over an hour in a panic. What the hell had happened in the operating room? Why was my arm so swollen? Why isn't anyone talking to me? It must have been bad if they had to put an IV in my compromised arm and one in my neck. I was drugged but alert and my mind raced with worst case scenario, and I could feel the adrenaline flooding my system. By the time they let my friends in, I was in meltdown and imagining the worst. A minute later the doctor was there telling me how well the surgery went and that the swelling was just temporary. The doctor was apologetic that she wasn't there when I woke up an hour prior, but it was the lack of communication from anyone which was the problem.

Health care professionals are under a grave misconception. They think you are still "out" when you are coming out of the anesthesia because patients are drugged and therefore they assume not conscious of their surroundings. In fact, you are not unaware but *super-aware*. You are completely helpless in the recovery room and feel like you are drowning. I have never felt more vulnerable than in those first few hours coming out of anesthesia. Without compassionate eyes and communication, terror is sure to set in. That the hospital staff and administration is unaware of this phenomenon and doesn't address it effectively is just neglect. They need to be the *most* compassionate and communicative in the recovery room.

Once in the regular hospital room I was on a morphine drip – not my drug of choice as it makes me way too fuzzy. I wanted to stay in the hospital just one night and had to negotiate with the nurses to get off the morphine and get them to give me Vicodin so I could go home the next day. You can't go home with a morphine drip. This hospital stay provided the least attentive nursing care I received throughout this whole process. Nurses are having to spend way too much time inputting data on a computer and not enough time with the patients. And once again it is clear being in a hospital without an advocate (friend, family member or hired outside nurse) is a not wise.

TIP: You need a personal advocate in a hospital. Do not think because you are in a hospital you are being taken care of and therefore do not need someone from your team there. You are most likely on some form of medication, often pain medication, and therefore not necessarily in your right mind. You absolutely need someone, especially right after surgery, to hear for you, be clear on the directions from the doctor, maybe get you something to eat or drink or an extra blanket, answer the phone, get your medicine and ask questions – always ask questions!

Dr. Hayden had to totally rebuild me from the inside as the anatomy had been completely torn underneath the implant. Without a "shelf" there was no place to anchor the implant which is why it was sinking. As a result I had a lot of healing to do internally. She also reduced the other side for symmetry.

The first week was rough. I slept sitting up and Vicodin was once again my salvation. It's been two weeks now. I'm healing and other than complete fatigue, which overtakes me without warning, I am doing well. My chest doesn't look like the one I had but it looks like it is on the road to one I can live with. Thank you Dr. Hayden.

TIP: Firm pillows help. This is even a great gift to bring to someone who is recovering. When recovering from surgery you sometimes need to elevate a certain body part in order to keep the pressure off of it.

My experience at Saint John's and particularly my horrific experience in the recovery room made me think once again about where our health care system has led us. As I was trying to figure out what to do about it a questionnaire arrived in the mail asking for my input regarding my stay at Saint John's, it was signed by the acting head of the hospital. I filled out the questionnaire but I also called his office and asked if I could take him out to lunch. I explained to the secretary that I had just had my second surgical procedure in a month at St. John's and that they indeed had a problem.

As it turned out I didn't have to actually go to lunch to get my point across. The head of the hospital had the head of nursing services call me to discuss my dissatisfaction and explain how negligent I thought they were in the recovery room and during my overnight stay. She appeared completely unaware of the problem and thanked me for my comments and promised to look into it.

July 2006. I saw Dr. Hayden and scheduled another surgery. The implant, while staying high on my chest, is still migrating under my arm when I lie down. She will have to go in and anchor it on the side and add the nipple. The quote for this additional surgery was originally $4,500 but now since the side is still not staying in place and needs more stitching the cost will be closer to $6,500. Once again, a reconstruction hasn't turned out like planned. It doesn't upset me as much, maybe because I see light at the end of the tunnel and the results so far are so much better and maybe because I know there are only two options – live with it or get it fixed. I just want to get it done.

July 27, 2006. Had surgery two days ago… five hours long… too tired to write about it.

July 28, 2006. The surgery on Tuesday took longer than expected. Dr. Hayden had to repair a muscle (a procedure called "vest over pants") in order to get the implant to hold, add the nipple and do a fat transfer on top of the implant so that it would look a bit more natural. Other than a bad episode of the shakes coming out of anesthesia once home it was fairly uneventful. I just felt full of drugs and tried to detox with lots of water.

And I have to report that my experience in the recovery room was what it should have been…attentive, professional and compassionate. I came to find out later Dr. Hayden read them the riot act so they watched me like a hawk. So like all construction projects it took longer and was over budget but I am grateful that it is done.

TIP: While you may feel fine in the recovery room and decide to go home it is possible for you to have a delayed reaction to the anesthetic. To have a bad reaction at home alone would be terrifying. After any ambulatory procedure, hospitals will require you to have someone to take you home, but will not necessarily mandate you have someone stay with you for the first 24 hours, but you always should. I admit I haven't always followed this advice in the past but that episode made me realize I need to in the future.

August was a month of healing. The fatigue was childlike. Suddenly I would have to go to sleep. I tried to make sure I wasn't in the car by myself when this happened. Finally, by the end of the month, I was feeling stronger, and having never been to Yellowstone I headed for Jackson Hole, Wyoming to the Grand Tetons ("great breasts" in French).

It was a wonderful week of clean air, sunshine, magnificent animals and even a full moon. At one point I was in Yellowstone Park and a herd of buffalo decided to cross the road and head toward the car. Their mass was something to be admired and respected. They came so close to my car I could have reached out and touched a huge bull. My first thought was...God just walked by.

October 4, 2006. Yesterday I met with Linda for tea. She has since had two chemo treatments and lost her hair so she showed up with a short brunette wig. Her beautiful face was shining and her blue eyes clear. She had the appearance of someone who was fasting. The short hair made her beauty even more obvious. We had only an hour and she explained how the chemo has been affecting her. So far she is not overcome with nausea and is trying to put on a few pounds so she won't be too thin when she is sure the chemo will hit her like a freight train. The steroid medicine the doctor is giving her is making her feel out of sorts so she is hoping it can be cut back but it is all day-by-day.

She told me how she had to face telling her six-year-old son she was ill and losing her hair, clearly wanting to do it "the best way," hoping that it was right. She tried to use humor. When her son said something was funny and they were both laughing, she said, "You know what, how funny is it that the grown-up medicine that mommy is taking is making mommy's hair fall out." Removing her baseball cap she showed her son her soon to be bald head. He continues to laugh, seeing only the absurdity in the situation. She assured him that it would come back when she was well.

Days later I went to the cosmetic pigmentation office in Beverly Hills to get the nipple tattooed. The technician took one look and told me she can't do it until the nipple is the right size; one that matches my natural nipple on the other side. I have to go back to Dr. Hayden to get the nipple reduced. Dr. Hayden's office told me how busy she is and there is no room on the schedule to fit me in. Will it ever be finished?

TIP: The new nipple has a tendency to shrink as it heals so while large when first made it will likely go down in size.

After being admittedly impatient with Dr. Hayden's staff ("She is too busy to see you before the end of the year") as my tolerance for further delay was thin, I got them to accommodate me in order to have the nipple reduced so that I can have it tattooed. I have to get this completed. Again, the process can really weigh you down.

November 9, 2006. Dr. Hayden reduces the nipple. She describes it as doing origami, Chinese paper sculpting. And when she is done it looks like the real thing...amazing. In a couple of weeks I can have it tattooed by a professional cosmetic tattoo artist so the color matches the other side.

TIP: The nipple can be made from tissue the surgeon has left at the site during reconstruction or from a skin graft or using AlloDerm®. The papule (the part that extends) is always made longer as it will shrink 50% over time so if this is larger than you want give it some time, 3-6 months, before you decide if it needs to be reduced.

The new nipple has no sensation but once tattooed it and my new breast looks real enough that when I show someone my breasts now they ask, "Which one is real?" The nipple has made it look authentic, no doubt about it. Confusion, faking them out, sleight of hand or should I say breast, is the best I can do. When I look at it in the mirror my breast no longer stares back blankly and I finally have symmetry. There is a nipple present. It is disarmed, unable to fire sensation, but it looks the part. It took four visits to the tattoo artist to get the color right.

TIP: After reconstruction (implant or tram flap) they can create a new nipple from your own tissue. Of course there won't be any feeling coming from this nipple but it can

make for a more symmetrical looking result. When the surgeon first makes the nipple it will be the color of your skin. Pigmentation is added by a tattoo technician so the skin matches the color of your other nipple. Or if you had a double mastectomy they would tattoo both. This isn't generally painful on the reconstructed side because there is no feeling. I chose not to have them touch the native side. There are businesses that specialize in this kind of cosmetic tattooing. Irradiated skin doesn't absorb the color or heal or respond the way non-irradiated skin does which is why you need someone familiar with tattooing a reconstructed breast site and not a standard tattoo parlor. And while insurance in many states is bound to pay for everything related to reconstruction you may still have a dispute on your hands with reimbursement when it comes to the tattooing.

7

Vigilance is the New Normal

Cancer is crisis in the true meaning of the (word in) Chinese... which is composed of two characters, one meaning danger, the other meaning opportunity.

– D. Spiegel, "Conserving Breasts and Relationships," *Health Psychology*

December 2006 and I am in Michigan for Christmas. I've decided I want a breast MRI since I haven't had one in 18 months. When I had my last mammogram they only did one side because of the implant.

Entering the office of Dr. Saha's, my oncology surgeon, is sobering. Any thought that I was somehow stronger or the exception to the rule disappears like air from a balloon. I am no different than the many others sitting in that waiting room. Although here for a check-up and the authorization to get an MRI, the memories of the crisis of two years ago fills me. Images of the hospital and feelings of sadness, the push towards acceptance, the sense of urgency, pain and tears come back as if no time had passed.

There is a privacy issue in the medical community which has attempted to be addressed by HIPAA laws but in all medical offices, as you are waiting to be seen by the doctor, you hear the murmurs throughout the office. Like elevator music it seeps into your consciousness. "I need to check your blood pressure," "Do we have your films," "When is your pre-op?" I wonder about the answers to all these questions and the consequences for other patients.

A force of nature, Dr. Saha walks in and it's like a wave hitting the shore. He is an extraordinary man and being in his office again makes me aware of his deeply spiritual side. Indian sculptures and photos of Jesus and proverbs from St. Francis line the walls. He aids in the cures but he knows God's will is paramount. And like a wave he will be on to the next patient as quickly as the tide is going out so I need to get to the point. I tell him, "I want an MRI." He asks when I last had one. I tell him, "A year and half ago when I had the surgery." He scolds me, "With a recurrence you need to have a bone scan, CAT scan and breast MRI every year not just a mammogram." Here I thought I was doing pretty well with my request for monitoring but, according to him, not well enough. He sets up the tests.

TIP: You will need "authorization" from your insurance company before you have this test otherwise there is a chance it won't be covered. It has to be requested by the doctor so make certain the doctor's office takes care of this and that you get confirmation of the authorization. Authorization does not guarantee payment by the insurance company but it is a necessary step.

TIP: There is a tendency in the medical community to hang on to standards of time when it comes to monitoring. While you can overdo testing (radiation is not harmless), if you feel something needs to be tested ask your doctor about it, especially if it is a non-invasive procedure like an ultrasound. The outcome impacts *you* so if you think you need to check something suspicious out, do it! A

mammogram equals the amount of normal radiation you would receive over the course of 3 months. A digital mammogram gives off less radiation but it also creates more false positive results. A full body scan is equal to the amount of radiation you would normally receive over the course of three years. Again you must weigh the risks and benefits.

A week later I have the bone scan and CT scan; both are done in doughnut hole machines. I need an IV for the bone scan. Once again the nurse takes my request for the "smallest needle necessary" as a personal slight and I have to actively persuade her to give me a small needle for the IV. She gets upset with me and walks out of the room. Two other nurses come in, wondering what the dust-up was about and finish the procedure. I can't resist and tell them that some people should be hairdressers and not be nurses and this woman is one of them. Don't let them bully you!

TIP: Ask the nurse to use the smallest possible IV needle that will allow for the rapid injection of the contrast. This isn't an operation where you will be under for hours – no need for a large needle. Same goes for a blood draw; always ask for the smallest possible needle that will not damage the blood cells. Nurses are often on automatic pilot and a butterfly needle is more expensive. Also post mastectomy they shouldn't draw blood or take your blood pressure on that side. If you've had a double mastectomy you don't have this option but should choose the side that has experienced less trauma.

I am scheduled to have the breast MRI the next evening. I have an anxiety-filled day absolutely dreading the test but when I show up the machine is broken and I have to come back the following week. In this case it was out of my hands and circumstances gave me another week, and when I did have it, I was mentally in a much better place.

The test came back "all clear." Breathe again.

TIP: Timing is something you need to be mindful of with every step. Often you won't be able to control it. You will be forced to do something before you are ready but if at all possible do it at a pace you can easily accept. Dr. Wayne Dyer writes about doing things along the path of least resistance. He compares it to the nursery rhyme. "Row, row, row your boat gently *down* the stream." Not up the stream. Take the path of least resistance when possible. It just makes it easier. When possible build some time between procedures and tests if you are uncomfortable and feeling rushed. Time allows for whole body integration. Integrating the experience helps you feel better prepared for the next step.

While I am in Michigan Dr. Saha and his wife, Luci, invite me and my nieces to their annual office Christmas party for his patients and staff. When we arrive the reception area of the oncology center is decorated for Christmas and long tables and chairs line every space. It appears as though there is enough food, from every country – Italian, Indian, and Polish – to feed a nation. It is abundant and heartwarming. I can feel the energy of the office change and I know this inclusive party, and the underlying feelings of goodness, will somehow permeate the office. This is an oncology center. It needs all the good energy it can get.

2007

March 22, 2007. My AOL account reminds me "I've got mail." The home page of AOL tells me Elizabeth Edwards' breast cancer has spread to the bone. It has made the leap from curable to incurable with that sentence. If it is just a lump and it hasn't microscopically traveled to other parts of your body there is a chance the surgeon got it all and it is curable. Once it is metastatic the whole ball game changes. Admittedly, the sad development sends a shudder through my system. Is the cancer lurking in the shadows? Hiding behind my liver? Dormant in my lung?

On the news that evening I am struck by her seemingly calm demeanor and her grace and gratitude for her support system. She mentions she has met so many people on the campaign trail who have told her stories of their own lives falling apart due to cancer and how sad she was for those who had to face it alone, or without resources, or without the best health care, or without insurance. She knows bad luck doesn't discriminate and she feels fortunate to have such tremendous support.

That said, she has Stage 4 metastatic breast cancer showing up in her bones – lucky is not a word I would use. Just last week her husband, John Edwards, when asked, "How is Elizabeth?" had replied, "She is *cancer free*." Of course he didn't know when she had her cracked rib X-rayed the test would tell a different story. It brings me back to *it isn't what is, it is only what we know to be true at the time.* "What is" is often not visible, like the wind.

They say the "cancer is back." Really? Or was it always there but just in a microscopic stage and we just don't have tests sensitive enough to pick it up? Everyone is so determined to declare victory in the form of the word "remission." Your cancer is in "remission" – those are the words you live for. The truth of the matter is we don't know where the cancer is. The medical experts cannot say for certain that there is no cancer present. All they can say is that according to the tests we have available in 2012 the cancer is not apparent. That is *all* they can say and that is the truth.

I think of four things when I hear about Elizabeth Edwards' cancer. The first is the devastation she felt in 1996 when her 16-year-old son Wade died and the physical and emotional stress that must have caused. It makes me suspicious again of the correlation between trauma and cancer.

Secondly, I think about her having been on a program of aggressive hormone therapy to get pregnant in her late 40s. Did either of these things contribute to her current condition? Once again I question how doctors can, in good conscience, offer fertility treatments to women in their 40s without insisting they at least follow the standard and get yearly mammograms. Elizabeth freely admits in her book *Saving Graces* that she hadn't had a mammogram in "too long, much too long." She implies that it was at least four years. "We moved to Washington four years ago and I never found a doctor there."

Most breast cancers are hormone receptive: 70 % of the cases. And women seeking fertility are prescribed extra hormones to help them get pregnant. Don't women realize this puts them possibly more at risk? Or do they realize it and ignore it not wanting to think that they are potentially putting their own health at risk for this primal urge to parent? Or does the desire and goal of getting pregnant blur the good judgment of all involved? Wouldn't vigilant breast screening be the very least these women are told they need? At the minimum they should be urged to follow the ACS standard of care of a yearly mammogram.

The third thought I have is that she first found a lump on October 21, 2004, while in the shower and here she is, March 2007, with Stage 4 cancer. That isn't a lot of time. By that date I have had breast cancer in my life for eight years. It makes me think how quickly some women need to adjust to a prognosis that is bleak.

And my final thought, unrelated to the cancer, is that her husband is the personification of ambition run amuck.

WHAT IS METASTATIC BREAST CANCER?

Metastatic breast cancer is not a different breast cancer. It is breast cancer that has traveled beyond the breast and can be detected in other parts of the body. The bone, brain, liver

and lung are the sites that are most common for what is termed a metastasis or distant recurrence of breast cancer. There is no cure for metastatic breast cancer but it can be treated. Even in those distant locations (lung, liver, bone, brain) it is still breast cancer.

2008

January 2008. So it is time once again for my yearly breast check-up. It seems to come around quicker every year. I do have a mass that I don't like in my right breast and a lump that was previously biopsied on my right side that is still there so I go into the exam with a certain amount of trepidation.

I am at Tower Imaging on Roxbury Drive in Beverly Hills. As I am waiting for my name to be called, I notice that the air is dense – filled with anxiety. A woman sits next to me and smiles nervously. "They could use a fountain in here." I tell her. "A little water flow to move the energy around." "Yeah. That would be good." She forces herself to take a deep breath.

I have both a mammogram and an ultrasound. The radiologists tell me both areas are benign. I feel like I dodged a bullet and go get some tea at the deli next door. In this case I had a bilateral mammogram but normally they only do the natural breast.

TIP: There are no official screening recommendations for women with a reconstructed breast (implant or tram) and a natural breast. Therefore, how you should be followed is something you should discuss with your breast surgeon. The individual nature of breast cancer has left us with no standard when it comes to monitoring after the disease. "Women with breast reconstruction on one side and a native breast on the other side are encouraged to undergo yearly surveillance mammography of the unaffected side. But there is no recommendation of what to do with the reconstructed side. It is clear that variations of practice

exist, and that we as physicians do not have a consistent way of following these women for local recurrence in their reconstructed breast," wrote Philip Barnsley of Dalhousie University in Nova Scotia in *Heal* magazine.

After hearing the good news I walked into a church in Beverly Hills, All Saints, and said a prayer. Church is a place where I feel closer to my mom. I couldn't call her and tell her the news, this was next best.

2009

July 2009. There are physical scars but they are fading – year by year. The internal emotional and psychological ones are much harder to heal and manage. How did this happen to me? I don't smoke, hardly drink, never did drugs, am not overweight and have no history of breast cancer. Without it being logical you are left wondering about what you have lost. And the loss is not just of your breast but of your good health and of what appeared to be the open road of your future. Yes, you work to transform it, overcome it, manage it, make the most of it but don't underestimate it: it is work. And then I remember "one in eight" and I realize that it isn't that it is illogical, quite the contrary, it is that we as a society have not fully accepted those facts and those odds, and prior to this experience I would have included myself in believing this is uncommon, especially in younger women.

Health condition: excellent...very good...good...fair. They say the breast cancer is gone. Does that mean on the health form when they ask about your health condition I get to check "excellent" like I used to? Does Lance Armstrong check "excellent"? I will have to ask him when I meet him. Or have I lost that label for good. Does it matter? Maybe. Like almost everything else some days it matters more than others.

I don't have children. I think of Elizabeth Edwards as I write this and of my friend Linda, and Jenny and Cathy and all the thousands of other women fighting cancer who have to look at their children as they do it. Not checking "excellent" when you have children who are counting on you can't be easy. It must weigh on you. I am sure it is as heavy a burden as the disease itself.

Part II

8

Men, Sex and Cancer

A woman is like a teabag, you never know how strong she is until you put her in hot water.

– Mae West

For many women breasts are a vital part of their sexual life. After all their very development was a signal that you were entering a different phase of your growth and are biologically and subconsciously linked with your sexual self. And breasts, from a sexual point of view, have the dual role of both being responsive and drawing response from the opposite sex.

Young women especially, ask the questions and do the worrying in the order of "My life? My breast? Can I still have a baby?" But for almost all women issues around sexuality and men and partnership are right there in the middle of the worry. How will they perceive me? Will he (or she) still love me? Will anyone love me? How do I feel sexy again? These are questions most women with a breast cancer diagnosis struggle with if you probe just a bit below the surface. While this can be especially concerning for single women, even women with steady partners struggle with the changes their bodies have undergone as a result of the cancer treatment, in addition to what natural aging brings, and no place more acutely than in the bedroom. And this is an issue that can well outlast the actual breast cancer treatment.

Intimacy can be fraught with ebbs and flows in the best of times. Add changes in your physical body, energy levels, mental focus and hormone fluctuations and it takes increased patience and understanding to make sexual intimacy a satisfying experience.

I first learned about sex by reading *Valley of the Dolls* (my mother's copy) when I was a teenager. By the way, Jacqueline Susann, its author, had a mastectomy in 1962 and died of breast cancer in 1974 at the age of 56. Susann and "The David Susskind Show" taught me almost everything I needed to know about sex.

As a girl, you could say, I was, "thrown into the deep end of the pool," when it comes to learning about the opposite sex. In the early 70s I went to The Peddie School, a New Jersey prep school that had just turned co-ed. At 13-years-old I was the only girl in almost all my classes. Taking biology when you are the only female in the room (including the teacher) will either make you confident or shy.

I matured sexually in the mid 70s right after the sexual revolution, in that window of time post birth control, pre-AIDS. In my adult life I always had confidence around sex and my sexuality but I admit breast cancer threw me. It made me question everything around men, dating, pleasure, partnership and sex. I had a long-term boyfriend when I first diagnosed but the obvious physical manifestations (the mastectomy and reconstruction) came when I was single. When I started dating again I would logically analyze the situation, think I had a handle on it and then the circumstances of possible sexual intimacy would arise and I couldn't help but panic a little. It rocked my femaleness like nothing else.

For a long time having had a diagnosis of cancer and a reconstructed breast and what it meant wasn't acceptable in my mind much less making anyone else feel at ease over it. Being able to compartmentalize would have come in handy during this phase of my life. If I could only "put it over there" but there was no there to put it. It entered the room before me and lingered like strong perfume. I couldn't escape it.

Prior to the surgery I could support my self-confidence with a little pampering. If it was a bad hair day I could go to the hair salon. If I just needed a mood lift I'd get my nails done or a massage and all the feminine energy would fill me and I would be ready to be with a man. But this seemed intractable. No amount of cute lingerie made it okay in my head. The physical numbness of one side of my chest made me feel cut off, as though my body wasn't fully integrated and I just wasn't myself.

Breast cancer had quite literally cut into my femininity, down to the bone. The complete acceptance of this I have still not conquered. It has become a practice continually requiring energy and compassion for myself. Some would say ignore it, get over it, move on...as a matter of fact I find myself saying that. But really, fully doing it is another story. To infuse what I consider now to be this brave part of my body, stitched together and artificially expanded with wholeness is a mental tug-of war. If you are struggling with this please know you aren't alone.

Slowly, in waves, it, my female self, has returned. I realize what I was feeling had as much to do with my energy and vitality as with my breast. The surgeries, change in my lymph system and the emotional burden of the disease had just depleted me. In this respect, I think any diagnosis of cancer can apply. You are fighting for your survival, anxious about the future and juggling your life. For women, at least all the ones I know, sex and sexuality are on the back burner until you are ready.

Also, breast cancer can make you have a lot of feelings that just aren't sexy. Anger, depression, sadness, a negative self-image, fatigue, lack of confidence and a sense of feeling overwhelmed can all contribute to your wanting to retreat rather than engage. And honestly, these feelings may make others want to retreat from you. You may be sending a lot of mixed messages. You need love but you are angry or sad. You want to be physically comforted but you are embarrassed with how you look so you withdraw. Fatigue and pain can make you irritable. Partners sometimes are at a loss too. Cancer throws everyone off their game.

And when your mental focus is on your health, it won't be on sex. All the topical creams in the world won't help if mentally you aren't ready because arousal and sexual interest happens first in the brain. All you have to do is look at the overwhelming recent popularity of the *Fifty Shades* series and realize women are craving mental escape. Those books resonated for so many because our mind is both our biggest ally and antagonist to having a satisfying sexual life.

Women in general engage in sex when they focus on it but getting ourselves to focus on it when our attention is elsewhere is the trick. We are easily distracted by the pressing concerns of life – children, work, our homes, shopping, our friends, our parents, our pets, etc. Everything needs to be *done*...then maybe we can think about it (which is why "vacation sex" is usually so much better). And when you are in a cancer battle rarely is everything *done* and your plate clear.

For me, it was men who helped me regain my balance. I chose very carefully and frankly was with men I knew would be accepting. Maybe that is why I had what I now call "my doctor period." I had never dated a doctor until I had breast cancer. Suddenly, handsome men with M.D.'s after their names became much more attractive to me. I was picking "safe" – they've seen it all – they won't be daunted. Anyone who didn't come with those credentials required more testing. I measured their character and level of tolerance for physical imperfection with conversational examples. Or I'd tell them about the breast cancer and analyze their facial expression. Did they just start tapping their foot? Was that a sudden twitch they developed?

So if you are worried about this hit to your femininity and lack of sexual interest realize a few things. First, of course you are. Secondly, it will take time to fully adjust. And thirdly, most women aren't interested in sex when they are using their energy for survival.

I have also come to know and appreciate that men are individuals too and there isn't a one size fits all reaction. Men can be more resilient and understanding than you may give them credit for, especially if they care for you. Sex, the hot variety, God-willing, is waiting and ready when you are.

So, bottom line, don't be hard on yourself if you are just not into it for a while. That said, choose carefully when it comes to romance, which you should do with or without cancer. One's heart is always worth giving and protecting. Maybe that cancer lesson has been especially clarifying. *Choose your mates as though your life depended upon it, because your time is your life, so it does.*

Some women I have talked to who have been through this with a steady sexual partner or husband say that their appreciation of the support they felt has made their sex life better with their partner, once they were feeling ready to reengage. Of course, breast cancer can also contribute to relationships ending and men and women moving on. Maybe this would have happened anyway, maybe not. Point being, you will never really know what triggers any separation. Like everything else breast cancer may bring, you can only deal with what is.

Cute lingerie may not solve the sex issue for you but nice bed clothes when you are feeling unsexy help. Invest in them like you would in a wig or a good bed. And I mean anything that makes you feel sexy if that is your mission. Sometimes a bit of luxury can go a long way, such as light cotton with a bit of rayon or a cashmere robe. Have it be comfortable with great fabrication and fit. And, like the sexy moves on "Sex and the City" you can sleep with a soft bra. Did you notice Sarah Jessica Parker almost always had TV sex with a bra on? Not that I am recommending you always wear a bra although not a bad idea if we are talking about a new partner and you aren't completely comfortable and it makes you feel less self-conscious – the killer of sexiness.

Yes, it is true, news flash – most men like breasts but they like the curves of a female body, a confident woman and soft skin more.

And if this partner is really right for you he will be more interested in your feeling good about yourself than complete nakedness. And always remember, experience usually brings wisdom and having sex with a wise woman is sexy.

TIP: Women who have been through chemotherapy and/or menopause may experience vaginal dryness. There are several lubricants on the market (Astroglide) that may help. Talk to your doctor about any discomfort during sex you are experiencing as they may be able to offer you some medications to alleviate the dryness.

FERTILITY AND CANCER

"My life, my breast, my ability to have children," that was the order of my concerns and I think I am not alone. My life. I must protect my life and do what I need to do to survive. My breast. I resisted even the possibility of a mastectomy knowing the detrimental effect of losing a seemingly defining body part would have on me. And then, almost in the same breath...my ability to have children. Is that going to be taken away too? I didn't have children at the time and thought when I was diagnosed children were still going to be part of my future. I didn't want cancer to make the decision for me. It was a good part of the reason I didn't go on tamoxifen when it was first recommended to me. Losing your fertility is a real fear and a reality that many younger cancer patients face.

Doctors are so focused on their goal of saving your life they don't often weigh the costs and consequences the way you do. But the powerful drive to reproduce and potential fear and sadness associated with that option abruptly being taken away can be a heavy burden, in addition to the disease.

The drugs, such as chemotherapy and tamoxifen, impact and almost always curtail fertility. That is one discussion if you have children already but quite another set of issues if you haven't yet had children and are still hopeful that they will be part of your future. For doctors to diminish this concern or worse ignore it in childbearing-age patients, is not to have a full understanding of the impact of the therapeutic protocol they may be suggesting. You may cure the patient but you may be crushing dreams that also go to the essence of who someone is and how they define themselves. When their image of their life included children, remaking that image and still having it feel successful and complete takes rethinking. It is as though the frame of your dream house was done and without warning a bulldozer came and knocked it down. But saving your life has to be the priority.

There are now organizations like www.fertilehope.com which can offer you help and hope around this issue. There is of course a lot of controversy regarding cancer and fertility treatment, especially when it is clear that the cancer you have is estrogen and/or progesterone receptive, in other words sensitive to hormones. With the advances in fertility options it may be possible to extract and save your eggs and preserve not end your chance of having a baby. However the risk incurred when adding more hormones to your system is something that needs to be considered very, very carefully.

Fertility treatments, while readily available, are still in their early stages of development. What is concerning about fertility treatment *for anyone* is that it isn't clear what effect these additional and usually high dose hormones have on a woman's risk of getting breast cancer. And what if a woman has an early stage breast cancer that hasn't yet been detected? Would these hormone boosts rev the engine of the cancer? Would pregnancy and the surge of estrogen feed tumor cells? In addition, the instant a woman gets pregnant she cannot be screened for breast cancer with a mammogram or MRI until she has not only gone through the pregnancy but has stopped breastfeeding. That can amount to many years and it is especially concerning with women over 40. *There have been no clear studies showing the risk of breast cancer is greater with fertility treatments but equally there have been no studies to refute the risk is not increased.* Left only to common sense, it would appear that you are indeed upping your chances of getting breast cancer. There is no evidence proving fertility treatments are harmless.

All that said, for many women having children is a mission and they will do just about anything to get pregnant. In many cases the cancer is temporary but the infertility is permanent – a distinction that should not be minimized in the effort to save a life but again, *saving a life has to be the priority.*

YOUNG WOMEN GET BREAST CANCER TOO

While age is a significant risk factor – the older you are the higher your risk – breast cancer in young women tends to be more aggressive and therefore an even more formidable threat. Approximately 11,000 women under the age of 40 are diagnosed with breast cancer every year in the U.S.

Problematic for the younger breast cancer patient is that often her concerns go unheard. "You are too young to get breast cancer" has been said to too many young women who indeed had the disease and precious time evaporated trying to get the right diagnosis. While breast cancer in young women is relatively uncommon, it is not impossible, far from it. Between the ages of 20 and 30 the chances are 1 in 2000, between the ages of 30 and 39 chances are 1 in 229, and between the ages of 40 and 49 the chances are 1 in 68.

One of the issues is when you are young, your breasts are denser (due to more connective tissue and fat) and therefore it is harder to detect by mammography if there is a problem. Now with digital mammography, radiologists can enhance the image making it somewhat easier to read. Still, early diagnosis in young women remains difficult.

There are so many factors that are different for a young patient: concerns about children, fertility, sexuality, body image, aggressive nature of tumors in younger women, husbands or the absence of one, mortality, a sense of unfairness and lack of support groups reflecting their age and circumstances. It is easy to be overwhelmed and depressed. Not only do you have this disease, it is hard to find anyone who can relate to you and your circumstances.

I admit I often thought, especially after the mastectomy, that I was glad I was at least 40 when this happened to me. I would have hated missing that carefree part of my life in my 20s and 30s worrying about breast cancer. I would have felt cheated and I imagine most young breast cancer patients feel that way too. It is understandable, as there is so much at stake and just when your future as an adult is being formulated. These patients need a lot of extra support as they often don't have the financial or emotional resources older patients might have.

HOW OFTEN SHOULD YOU GET SCREENED?

Because 70% of breast cancers are hormone receptive (ER and PR positive) it would make sense for tumors to grow more aggressively when you have more hormones in your system. While the standard has been to have a baseline mammogram at age 40 (according to the ACS), if you have a family history or any concern, get a screening mammogram earlier. I had my first one at 18 when something suspicious showed up under my arm. It proved to be nothing but that experience made me more vigilant about my breast health.

The new, and in my view misleading and damaging Preventative Task Force guidelines of 2009 stipulating you should get your first mammogram at age 50, should make younger patients want to cry out, "Are you crazy?" In my view the real damage caused by these guidelines is to reinforce the myth that somehow you are "safe" from this disease until you turn 50. The reality is women lose their life in their 20s, 30s and 40s because of breast cancer every single day.

TIP: The Young Survival Coalition is a group that supports young breast cancer patients.

TIP: You are never too young to get breast cancer. Have anything suspicious checked out by a qualified physician.

MEN ARE NOT EXEMPT

For everyone who thinks breast cancer is just a woman's disease, I've got news for you. Men get breast cancer too and in higher numbers than most people, even people familiar with this fact, realize.

According to the American Cancer Society, in 2011 there were 2,140 cases of male breast cancer diagnosed in the U.S. and 450 deaths. Of course men are not getting screened for this disease the way women are and there is considerable misinformation, denial and embarrassment around the disease for men making early diagnosis less likely.

According to the American Cancer Society these are the known risk factors:

Aging

Men with breast cancer average about 67 years old at the time of diagnosis.

Family history of breast cancer

About 20% of men with breast cancer have a close male or female relative with the disease.

Inherited gene mutations

BRCA1 and BRAC2 gene mutations apply. Approximately 10% of all breast cancer cases in men are attributed to these gene mutations. There is also a gene mutation called CHEK 2 which may be responsible for some male breast cancers.

Klinefelter syndrome

This is a congenital disease which affects 1 out of 1000 men. Normally men have a single X chromosome along with their Y chromosome while women have two X chromosomes. Men with this condition have more than one X chromosome (sometimes as many as 4). This causes their testicles to be smaller than usual and for them to produce non-functioning sperm cells, making them infertile. Compared with other men they have lower levels of androgens (male hormones) and more estrogens (female hormones). For this reason they often develop gynecomastia (benign male breast growth).

Radiation exposure

A man whose chest area has been exposed to radiation (usually for treatment of cancer inside the chest, such as Hodgkin's lymphoma) has an increased risk of developing breast cancer.

Alcohol

Heavy alcohol intake increases the risk of breast cancer in men.

Liver disease

Men with severe liver disease such as cirrhosis of the liver have relatively low levels of androgen activity and higher estrogen levels. Therefore this may increase the risk of developing gynecomastia and breast cancer.

Estrogen-related drugs or treatment

Physical inactivity or obesity

Obesity raises estrogen levels.

9

The Words, the Consequences

I've learned that people will forget what you said, people will forget what you did, but people will never forget how you made them feel.
– Maya Angelou

WHAT DO YOU SAY TO SOMEONE THAT HAS BEEN DIAGNOSED WITH CANCER?

"*I have breast cancer.*" No one wants to have a conversation that starts this way. I remember the experience of telling almost every important person in my life. It tends to be a struggle both for the person confiding the information and the person it is being shared with. Telling those you love, or even relative strangers, can be difficult. Appropriate honesty and compassion need to be at work and yet many are left speechless or worse, offering words that don't validate the situation.

I would say first, as the patient, to have no expectations because in these moments of crisis very few people will be able to offer you the comfort you need and/or want. We haven't been taught to react to such uncertain circumstances. Often people are quick to say, "Everything is going to be all right." Really? How do they know that? Of course they don't. They want things to be fine, they want to reassure you, so they speak from that place.

Fact is, they don't know what is going to happen and neither do you. Others show distance, appearing almost disinterested, when in fact they are likely just lost, having no idea what you need and are afraid of their own emotions around illness and lack of control. And yet others want to take over because they themselves can't accept the fact that you are sick. They are going to "fix it."

One woman distraught over having lost her hair heard a friend say, "I don't think it would bother me to lose my hair." Well, it bothered her and having a friend take an opposite hypothetical view didn't help. Fact is, until you walk in the shoes of a cancer patient you really have no idea what you will do or not do or how you will feel about it.

What most of the cancer patients I have spoken with want to hear first and foremost is validation that the situation is indeed rotten. That while you hopefully will get well, the diagnosis is terrible and what you are faced with won't be easy. Acknowledgment of the bad news is validating. That said, leaving it at that isn't helpful.

I think one of the best things you can say if you want to offer support is along the lines of, "I've always admired your... (add what's true... courage, strength, humor, willfulness, etc.) When you did such and such, it inspired me. This cancer will test you but I have witnessed your strength and resourcefulness. You can fight this." If you will be actively involved in the process as a friend or a caretaker then you can express your support. If not, then pledging prayers and good thoughts might be appropriate.

WHAT IS A HUSBAND, FATHER, FRIEND, SON, AND BROTHER TO DO? WHAT ABOUT ANYONE WHO IS THE CAREGIVER?

When a woman gets breast cancer she feels attacked and vulnerable. She may very well feel betrayed by her own body. Her need for security, comfort and acceptance soars. The men in her life

– partners, dads, brothers, friends, or even co-workers – can offer enormous support if they choose not to retreat. Embarrassment, lack of control and the feeling of not wanting to pry or be invasive can make a man go silent. Fellows, I assure you this is no time to be invisible – we need your presence and strength.

As a patient you are under stress and often overwhelmed, making it hard to draw on your own reserves. You are just plain tired. The vitality and confidence of others around you can be of great comfort. You may be telling yourself, "It is going to be okay" and "I am going to get through this" but your voice may be weakening with each treatment and diagnosis. Hearing words of encouragement from family members and friends you trust while still validating the difficulty can go a long way toward bolstering your resolve to go on.

In my experience when men can't fix something rather than "fail" would rather not try in the first place and withdraw. Many a husband has found refuge in a man's den: the garage, office, bar or basement. It is true that the men in your life are not going to be able to "slay this dragon" for you but the way they stand by you fortifies your ability to fight on. It is important that they know their presence and strength is critical to you. Fully appreciating what they do for you and expressing it as best you can, will fuel them to be more supportive. Try a positive approach as criticism will only shut them down further. What they need to know is a phone call, a hug, flowers, a bowl of chicken soup, a card, a book, a favorite CD, an invitation to walk in the park or a ride to the ice cream store – are all simple expressions of care and comfort that can make a difference.

Having a discussion upfront about what the partner in your life will be able to do for you may be in order. Will he or won't he interface with the doctor, do the grocery shopping, take care of the kids, inform your parents or others who are having a hard time coping with your diagnosis or be the record keeper or the insurance liaison? This isn't to abdicate your involvement but to outline what would be helpful to you. Having breast cancer brings up issues of trusting your own body but you still want to be able to trust someone else and that is why it is important to have open and honest communication about what appropriate role a partner can and will play.

If a man were to say to a doctor, with all good intentions of trying to protect his wife or partner, "Give it to me straight doc, but don't tell her," it sets up an invisible barrier, a situation where one person has information the other doesn't, which can lead to misunderstandings. Some women don't want to know every prognosis and are relieved to have someone shoulder the information. Others would rather know every detail. What is important is that the woman decides how it should be handled; whatever happens is with her full acknowledgement and permission. Often I have heard the refrain, "he is my rock," referring to a partner who has chosen to stand by and be fully present during this trying time with her. Lucky girl!

Many women go through this without partners and some women are going through this with partners who are not able to give in a nurturing way. It is most important that you reach out to them. As a friend your small gesture of support or encouragement will be remembered long after the sickness has passed.

The definition of "to witness" is to have knowledge of a firsthand account of events. This person, the one who goes to doctor appointments, stands at the side of your bed, makes sure you are getting the right medicine, brings food and provides comfort is of utmost importance. Choose them carefully. Again, it is up to you.

WHAT CAN YOU SAY TO THE CHILDREN OF A MOTHER WHO HAS BREAST CANCER?

In the movie *Terms of Endearment*, the character Debra Winger played is dying of breast cancer and has to say good-bye to her young children. I remember her trying her best to prepare her children for what was to come. She clearly wasn't going to be there anymore physically but was desperate to have her mothering influences live on. In her deep, throaty voice, Debra Winger showed all the fatigue of a breast cancer patient yet she is still young and spiritually vibrant. It looks wrong. Like too many real women with much to live for, she is too young to die. As she imparted her last words of motherly wisdom there wasn't a dry eye in the house. There isn't anything much more heart-wrenching than a mother having to say good-bye to her young children.

All cancer is not alike and all breast cancer is not alike, so a lot depends on the diagnosis and prognosis of the patient. But even the threat of losing a parent and or seeing one with diminished capacity, even if it is only temporary, can be scary to a child. Children want their parents to be strong and shield them. Losing that protection in any way can certainly undermine one's sense of security in the world.

So what do you say to the children? I asked some of the affected women who do have children and this is what they said. First, children know something is wrong. Hiding it only makes it feel like your sickness has something to do with them. And secondly, you can't protect them from reality but you can soften the impact.

According to Kathleen Mojas, Ph.D., a psychologist in Beverly Hills, "What is important is that children be allowed to express their feelings and be heard. Being told to 'be strong' for a parent can short-circuit the child's ability to process the experience."

The powerful subconscious has no sense of time. Therefore trauma experienced many years' prior lives in the subconscious as though it just happened. Even as adults, childhood trauma can haunt our lives and our dreams and trap us into behavior that is destructive and self-defeating. And the worst part is without professional treatment we can't access the source and really heal the wound. Dr. Mojas has had great results with EMDR (Eye Movement Desensitization and Reprocessing), a technique that helps the brain reprogram the trauma so that it takes its proper place in the past and loses the hold over us. This technique has been proven to be helpful in adults and children. For children who have gone through the sickness or death of a parent professional treatment may be beneficial in dealing with the source of the anxiety and sadness.

Unfortunately, the scene of a young mother dying in *Terms of Endearment* plays out all over the world for real with children saying good-bye too early to mothers stricken down too young. The children are usually rendered speechless, not even knowing what to ask or say as the whole concept of being left as a child is unnatural.

Again this is especially hard on mothers with young children and makes getting breast cancer at a young age, where the cancer can be more aggressive, that much more tragic. More often than not, cancer not only affects an individual but an entire family and frequently it is the young children who have to live with the devastating fallout from this disease...growing up without a parent.

My experience of children losing a young mother and the farewell that must take place was watching my nieces say goodbye to their mom. It was renal cancer, not breast cancer, which took her life but the dying is much the same. The morphine or other heavy duty pain medicine coursing through a dying person's system can make them say things and even do things that can hurt those watching them die. It happened to me when my mom died and it happened to my nieces as my 50-year-old sister-in-law was ill. I tried to protect them from her harsh drug, induced words but there were some occasions when the words were already spoken before I could head it off.

One day, about a week before my sister-in law Peggy died, her daughter, 14-year-old Monica, came upstairs with a cup of tea for her mother, such a gesture of kindness. Peggy looked at her, looked at the tea and out of the blue said, in an angry tone, "Monica Lynn, don't you lie to me." Monica looked crushed and confused. She looked at me for an explanation. She hadn't even said anything and this was Peggy's greeting to her. Somewhere, in the recesses of Peggy's mind, there was an unresolved issue and the morphine freed her to speak. I was standing there and able to diffuse it somewhat telling Monica she didn't mean it, that the drugs were making her a little crazy but the words were out and therefore had life. Like escapees from Pandora's Box, words not based in reality but would become reality for a child already hurting.

TIP: Be aware that pain medication can make people say things they wouldn't normally say and in a tone they wouldn't generally use. This can be very hard on caretakers. The patient will reach back to an old conversation or set of feelings unresolved and then speak about them, sometimes in an unkind voice. They know not what they say but if you are the recipient, and this person is your mother or father, the words can be searing. As an adult hopefully you will have an understanding of the power of the drugs and know that what they are saying is not meant to hurt you. But a child doesn't have this kind of perspective and these moments of good-bye can be cemented into the consciousness making the hurtful feelings hard to overcome and process.

My experience with this kind of situation came about a month prior to my own mom's death. They had her on heavy doses of morphine. I had been in the hospital all day with her and this had been going on for weeks. I was in that stage when you are on automatic pilot, numb, just trying to get though the crisis. My cousin Joe came by the hospital after work to see her. As he was sitting in the chair, still in his work clothes, making small talk, my mom, in a drug altered state, suddenly started yelling and criticizing me out of the blue. It was clearly out of context and I knew Joe felt terrible not only for my mom but for me, never having seen her act this way before. And even with my full knowledge that it was drug-induced, the memory lives.

If all you want to do is comfort a parent and they are hostile back it can be devastating, especially for children. Monitor this if you are the adult in charge. And of course if you are reading this and know that in your future you may very well be on a lot of pain medication speak about it in advance and assure people how you really feel about them. A pro active approach will go a long way towards healing any misunderstanding that may come about as a result of the drugs. It is never too early to tell someone you love them and appreciate them. If you need the words it could go something like this...

"I have a difficult road ahead of me. I may not be myself for part of this as I am likely going to need powerful, mind-altering drugs to get though it which may make me say and do things I am not fully conscious of. I want you to know, before this begins, that I love you and am grateful for your care and concern. Forgive me if I say anything to hurt you as I am being treated. It isn't how I feel in my heart. Do you understand me?"

Allow for dialogue around this. Your act of vulnerability may give permission to others to act likewise. You may be surprised by the openness it creates and it may turn out to be a significant and cherished conversation. Yes, it all takes courage.

CONSEQUENCES OF SURGERY AND TREATMENT

You may know of some of the obvious and more talked-about side effects of surgery and treatment for breast cancer: losing one's hair, sexual side effects, losing a breast, scars, both physical and emotional. But there may be some unintended consequences that are somewhat unforeseen that may also affect you. These are quality of life issues that can have an impact long after the original cancer has been treated.

Weakness

With surgery, especially after a mastectomy, you may find some weakness and numbness in that arm or side. This may affect your mobility and it may affect your balance and relative strength. If prior to surgery you had nearly equal strength on your left and right side, you may find diminished strength on the compromised side. The repercussions of this may not be fully evident until you resume your normal lifestyle and can be especially troubling if at one time you were athletic and return to sports.

Lymphedema

Lymphedema is a condition that is brought on by the accumulation of lymphatic fluid. Lymphedema is a real concern in breast cancer treatment especially if it involved the sampling or near total removal of lymph nodes. Your risk of developing lymphedema should be discussed with your doctor early on in your treatment so that you can be prepared to do whatever possible to avoid or mitigate the condition. Unfortunately despite your best efforts, it cannot always be completely prevented.

Lymphedema is of significant concern, not just for medical reasons; there is also the factor of self-image. Having a swollen extremity can be embarrassing, in addition to the discomfort – the heaviness, numbness and fullness associated with a lymphedematous extremity. Certainly enough reasons to do what you can to avoid this condition if at all possible.

The lymph system is a one-way filtration system in the body that allows lymph (fluid) to be transported through the body, flow into the central circulation and be ultimately expelled by the kidneys. The lymph vessels have the ability to pump to the lymph collectors and then to the lymph nodes. If this system is working properly there is a constant removal of lymph. If this is disrupted or compromised, the valves, rather than pumping, stay in an open position and fluid does not disperse in a normal way. The result is swelling of arm(s) and or leg(s). Any swelling should be brought to the attention of your doctor immediately.

A minor case of lymphedema can be uncomfortable – a feeling of fullness or heaviness. In more severe cases there can be extreme swelling and discomfort which if left untreated could lead to skin breakdown, inflammation, and even infection where skin can become hot and red and is often accompanied by a fever, a condition called cellulitis. This in turn can potentially lead to sepsis – a life-threatening condition.

While we all generally have similar lymph systems, everyone's lymph system is unique to them – the size of the nodes, number and capacity are all individual and therefore reactions to lymph node surgery, radiation and chemotherapy will also differ. Not everyone will develop lymphedema and it may come and go depending on an individual's exercise level, weight, temperature or even air travel, brought on by pressurized cabins.

If you do have to contend with lymphedema it can be managed and many of the symptoms can be reversed with treatment. According to Mary Rosenberg, P.T., a lymphedema specialist and owner of the Hollywood Physical Therapy Associates, Hollywood, California, "Lymphedema is a quality of life issue and one that is often forgotten about until after the cancer has been diagnosed and treated. The lymphatic system is a one-way transport system. With fluid build-up you have essentially a 'road block' and the physical therapist has to find new pathways for you. With the use of specialized compression bandages, massage and movement, lymphedema can be treated."

Mary has some tips for you to keep in mind from the *Lymphedema Information Booklet*.

1) Don't assume medical caretakers know you are at risk for this. Do not allow them to use a blood pressure cuff on the compromised arm.
2) Same for blood draws. Do not let them draw blood from your compromised arm. If you have had a double

mastectomy choose the side that has had the least amount of trauma.

3) With a blood draw ask for a butterfly needle or the smallest needle possible that will not alter the lab results. Butterflies are more expensive and won't always automatically be offered.
4) Know that the greater the blood flow, the greater the lymph production. While light exercise may be good, overdoing it may bring on more swelling.
5) If you have lymphedema you should be fitted for special garments in order for you to exercise more safely.
6) Consider lymph drainage massage by a specialist.
7) Other symptoms can include swelling of the hand, a pulling on the neck or an almost wooden sensation in the arm. These symptoms should be brought to the attention of your doctor immediately.
8) When traveling don't lift heavy luggage or wear constrictive clothes. Do move around on long flights, elevate the arm as much as possible and stay away from caffeinated beverages.
9) There are emotional consequences to lymphedema for some women. The cosmetic issue should not be underestimated and professional psychological help may be required.

CLINICAL TRIALS – CREATING THE DATA THAT MAKES TREATMENT POSSIBLE

A clinical trial is a controlled sampling of patients who agree to be part of a specific study for a certain period of time. Clinical trials are designed to scientifically assess the effectiveness of a treatment or drug. However, more or cutting edge is not always better. As Dr. Mehmet Oz says, "The latest thing isn't always the greatest thing."

When you are given heart-stopping news it makes perfect sense that you might seek out experimental treatment hoping for the wonder drug. While this is a natural reaction, being part of a clinical trial is just that...a clinical trial. The medical experts running the clinical trial have assumptions they are trying to prove but perhaps no hard evidence. The clinical trial is what they hope is going to prove their theory, the evidence they need to move forward. You may feel you have little choice but to enter a clinical trial, that you have to do everything possible, even if it means putting yourself at risk in an experimental study. The self-imposed desire to survive and do all you can in addition to the sometimes perceived pressure from friends and family can be enormous. But being part of a clinical trial is an individual decision with potentially major repercussions.

High dose chemotherapy (HDC) with bone marrow or stem cell transplant for the treatment of breast cancer sounds like a good idea (let's kill it all and replace with new cells) but in actuality there is no scientific evidence to support its effectiveness at this time. As the NBCC reports, 30,000 women were given this treatment and yet the numbers show it was no more effective than regular chemotherapy. The women who opted to have bone marrow treatment are beyond brave. With this choice they face many side effects – nerve damage, hearing loss, possible weeks of isolation, much higher risks of infections and sometimes death.

Since many clinical trials are ongoing, with some generating a lot of enthusiasm due to their *potential*, doctors sometimes recommend treatment based on the fact of the trial's existence and not on the fact that the data may or may not be compelling. It is true that without clinical trials we wouldn't have the drugs and advancements we currently have in place. Every drug on the market was in, at one time, a clinical trial. Many courageous women have endured much, resulting in the current protocols available today. Still, it isn't for everyone.

Clinical trial success for doctors and researchers often means that this or that drug will add days or at the most months to a life. What they are offering may or may not be enough for you given the downside. The doctors and the drug companies are in a race to be able to string enough drugs together that are relatively successful to add years to life spans but in the process it is measured in days.

A drug that adds an extra month is considered a success. However, doctors need to be ever mindful that their single biggest priority is you, the patient before them, and not getting research for their drug trials, no matter how pressing the need. Doctors need to ask themselves if this were their mother, sister or wife would they encourage participation for the sake of science?

And maybe we need to focus more on the successes. Studies around long-term survival are few. Dr. Susan Love was inspired by a colleague who suggested that success was worth studying and through her research foundation is now examining long-term survival. This idea germinated from a study from World War II, when they started studying the airplanes that stayed in the air rather than just the ones that fell from the sky.

If you are interested in being part of a clinical trial the National Cancer Institute has important information on its website or you can call 1-800-4 Cancer. It is vital you understand that being in a clinical trial does not guarantee you will get the new drug or therapy. It is possible you could end up in the "control group," the group used to measure the effectiveness of the new treatment against. The control group does not get the new drug or therapy.

ALTERNATIVE MEDICINE

Doctors in America are licensed by the government. The doctors are only allowed to recommend treatment that the FDA (Food and Drug Administration) approves. Doctors and the FDA are lobbied intensely by the pharmaceutical industries with multiple salespeople courting each doctor. Sometimes doctors actually get cash payments (so called discounts) paid directly to them from the drug companies for prescribing their drugs. Drug companies are in the business of making money and paying shareholders. They are for-profit companies. I don't know of any intentionally nonprofit drug companies. Herceptin, for instance, a drug used for aggressive breast cancer, is a billion dollar *a year* business. The more expensive the drug and the greater the demand, the more the drug company makes.

Alternative treatments and certainly preventative care do not have a lobby and their profit has never really been measured. Perhaps no one is promoting them and there are no clinical trials around them because there is not sufficient profit, not because they don't or wouldn't work: we just don't know. We will never know unless they are tested but without a profit incentive that is not going to happen in the current system.

Again, 17% of our Gross National Product is spent on health care. To think that the protocols are not linked to profit motive is naïve. The whole health structure is oriented around the treatment of disease. That is the core profit center, not prevention or eradication.

If you are doing anything which is considered "alternative" you should make your doctors aware of your decisions. That includes any herbal supplements or vitamin regimes since they may cause possible adverse reactions with your treatment.

10

Facts, Possible Causes and Action

Give it to me straight, doc.

–Humphrey Bogart

THESE ARE THE FACTS:

The American Cancer Society estimates that U.S. women have a 1 in 8 chance of developing invasive breast cancer in their lifetime. One in 25 will die of it.

Approximately 3.3 million women in the U.S. are currently living with breast cancer. 2.3 million women have been diagnosed and an estimated 1 million do not yet know they have the disease.

In 2011, 288,130 women were diagnosed with breast cancer (invasive and non-invasive).

The average age of getting breast cancer is 61years of age.

Peak age of getting breast cancer is 75-79 years of age.

95% of breast cancers are in women 40 and older.

Age 40 is an *arbitrary* marker for screening.

One mammogram is equal to about 3 months of normal radiation.

50,430 women under 50 were diagnosed in 2011 with invasive breast cancer. There were approximately 2,830 breast cancer deaths of women under 45 in 2007. (One of the primary reasons for writing this book is that breast cancer in young women is particularly deadly and all too often has gone misdiagnosed because women are young and therefore the symptoms are either missed or dismissed.)

Your risk of developing breast cancer between the ages of 30-40 is 1 in 252.

There is no known way to prevent breast cancer.

Breast density is a risk factor due to the fact it can make it harder to detect a problem on a mammogram.

Breast cancer is the second leading cause of death for women in the U.S. (after lung cancer). Approximately 39,520 women died from the disease in 2011. Breast cancer is the leading cause of death for U.S. women between the ages of 20 and 59, and the leading cause of death for women worldwide.

There were approximately 57,650 cases of non-invasive breast cancer diagnosed in the U.S. in 2011 according to the ACS.

Approximately 12% of women diagnosed with invasive breast cancer die from the disease within five years; at ten years 20% will have died. The most recent available studies show that 40% of all women diagnosed with invasive breast cancer died from the disease within 20 years. (This 20 year survival statistic was obtained by studying women diagnosed with breast cancer 20-years ago. It is impossible to know what the 20 year breast cancer survival rate will be for women diagnosed today.)

Older women are much more likely to get breast cancer than younger women. Most breast cancers – about 77% – occur in women ages 50 and older. About 5% of all breast cancer cases occur in women under the age of 40. However, younger women who get breast cancer have a lower survival rate than older women who get breast cancer.

All women are at risk for breast cancer. About 90% of women who develop breast cancer do not have a family history of the disease.

Mammography screening does not prevent or cure breast cancer. It is estimated breast cancer tumors can exist six to ten years before they grow large enough to be detected by mammography. In addition, mammography is less effective in younger women than in older women due to the density (high-fat ratio) of their breasts. Fat and connective tissue and tumors show up as white on an X-ray making them hard to distinguish.

In Saudi Arabia you generally need your husband's permission to get a mammogram.

Around the globe this year there will be more than 1.3 million breast cancers diagnosed and over 460,000 people will die of the disease.

Men get breast cancer too. In 2011, approximately 450 men in the U.S. died from the disease. One in five of those men have a relative (daughter, sister, and mother) with breast cancer.

If you are a woman between the ages of 50-59 you have a 1 in 37 chance of getting breast cancer.

WHAT CAUSES BREAST CANCER?

Fact is no one knows. The experts know what might put you at higher risk for getting it but they don't know the trigger. Where and why does the controlled cell become the uncontrolled one? Is it one trigger or a convergence of triggers? And why in some people and not others? Age, obesity, family history – they all raise your risk but there is no advanced test to determine if you will *definitely* get breast cancer. So we can speculate as to what might have an impact...genetic history, age, environment, diet, trauma, alcohol, smoking, latent or no pregnancy but no one can give you an individual definitive answer. And while we currently put all breast cancers under the banner of breast cancer, all breast cancers are not alike and therefore may very well have different etiologies. And since everyone is an individual the reality is no two people have the exact same disease.

Age

As you age, your risk of getting breast cancer increases. The majority of breast cancer happens in people over 50.

Hormone Replacement Therapy

Hormone Replacement Therapy (HRT) was standard of care for post menopausal women in America for years. Some forms of hormone replacement therapy are now considered to increase your risk of heart disease and breast cancer especially if is taken long term. Talk with your doctor about HRT and ask questions of the implications.

Smoking

This is a known carcinogen and one that raises your risk of getting breast and lung cancer.

Obesity and Lack of Exercise

Both are factors that increase your chances of getting breast cancer. Fat cells can produce and store estrogen, again raising the possibility that higher hormone levels may contribute to higher breast cancer risk.

Environmental Factors

Some chemicals in our air, food and water are known carcinogens. High toxicity levels are linked to cancer. Cosmic radiation in aircraft is also an area of concern.

Lack of Pregnancy or Late Pregnancy

Pregnancy changes the architecture of the breast. Studies indicate that late pregnancy or lack of pregnancy can increase your risk.

Alcohol

There is a definite link between alcohol consumption and breast cancer, according to the ACS. The more alcohol you drink the higher your risk.

Family History

Genetics certainly play a prominent role in terms of risk factors but the experts can't say it causes cancer, just predisposes you to it.

Some try to evaluate risk based on the "Gail model," named for Dr. Gail, the biostatistician who created it. Much of this information was collected from Caucasian women and due to this fact may not accurately calculate the risk to African American woman. And while the Gail model is based on known risk factors, many women who have breast cancer don't possess any known breast cancer risk. Again the failure of the medical community to exact a "breast cancer equation" that applies to all women proves breast cancer is an individual and somewhat mysterious disease.

IS THERE AN EMOTIONAL COMPONENT? TRAUMA AND HEARTBREAK

In the 21st Century I imagine the emotional component of one's life related to cancer will be studied. How does it contribute to your body's internal environment that may allow the cancer to grow? There are sure to be more studies about the immune response to cancer and while the therapies will get more targeted the treatments may start to take into account the whole person, including what has gone on and is going on emotionally for the individual.

Two circumstances that certainly have a detrimental effect on us as people – trauma and heartbreak – have not been studied widely, if at all, and yet my own personal experience makes me wonder if there is a link. Clearly we all process our experience and emotions differently. To what degree, if any, our emotional history has an impact on our medical history will I believe be left to future generations to determine more fully.

Trauma

Does trauma cause cancer or change our immune response? Of course we don't know. However, I am always struck by the coincidence of high stress or trauma and cancer. Again I can only speak from personal experience and my instincts tell me there is some sort of connection.

In 1973 I survived an attempted rape in my bathroom dormitory at Franklin and Marshall College. It was my freshman year, I had just turned 18, and up until that point, college had been a dream come true. I had made new friends, had a terrific roommate, a new wonderful boyfriend and was doing great academically. That night, in November 1973, the weekend before Thanksgiving, my life changed forever.

I came home from a Saturday night date at 2:00 in the morning. My boyfriend dropped me off at my dorm. I changed into a football jersey for sleeping and with my toiletries headed towards the bathrooms, which were in the center of the hall. As I was washing my face in the sink a man came from behind me, put his hand over my mouth, slammed me into his chest and dragged me to the floor. I never saw his face just his dark wool cap in the mirror.

It took everything in me to hold myself up with my left arm. To this day, I can still feel what the cold linoleum felt like under my left hand. He was very strong and tried to flip me over on my back but my left arm held. The force of his right hand on my face was crushing. My only thought was, "there is no way this guy is going to rape me." He said, "Take your panties off or I'll kill you and I'm not kidding." His grip pushed on my teeth and crushed my face. And then I felt part of his right ring finger was in my mouth. I bite his finger so hard I know I nearly bit it off.

In pain, he moved his hand off my mouth and I started to scream. Nervous that he was going to get caught, as the bathroom was located in the middle of the dorm hall, the coward fled. On his way out he grabbed the side of my underwear and ripped them from my body and left them there. He ran out of the bathroom, down the hall and out the back door into the park behind the dorm. I got up and, in shock, checked my teeth and face in the mirror since he had kept such a grip on me I thought for sure my teeth would fall out. They didn't, thank God. I went to the campus security phone in the hall and called security. The girls from my hall stood in their doorways in their nightclothes, awakened by screams, confused as to what had just happened. He was never identified and got away with it. I had a black eye from the force of his grip and an emotional imprint that has never completely left. I walked into the bathroom that night one girl and walked out another.

My breast cancer was on my left side. A direct line from my left hand, up my arm and to a spot right over my heart. Maybe it is a coincidence, maybe not. My own personal opinion is that cancer and trauma are somehow, in some cases, linked. I will feel this way until someone proves the contrary.

Heartbreak

Does our emotional life impact our health? Does heartbreak, and I don't just mean romantic heartbreak but deep sadness that can come from a variety of sources, reorganize our DNA? Grief, sorrow, sadness, stress – what is the impact on one's health? We have heard about people dying from a broken heart so maybe the impact of profound grief is more systemic than we currently recognize. It is true breasts make their own hormones. And we know that hormones are related to emotional bonding and certainly to sexual response. There seem to be many studies related to drug therapies but what about studies that explore the link between emotional distress and cancer. Is there a correlation?

YOU DON'T HAVE CANCER BUT YOU ARE WORRIED. WHAT CAN YOU DO?

First know how to examine your own breasts with breast self-examination. If you know what is normal for you then when an abnormal feeling comes up you have a better chance of recognizing it.

Breast Self Examination (BSE) and Knowing Your Body

Breast self-examination is important as I want to stress breast cancer usually does not cause pain in its early stages. You are the expert on your body. Recognizing the changes which may indicate there is a problem is essential. What is important here is that you become familiar with what is normal *for you*. However, *any abnormality* should be pointed out to a breast doctor and monitored and perhaps tested to make sure it isn't cancer. Too many women have felt lumps that weren't tested and proved to be a problem. The lack of pain makes it hard to know what is dangerous and what isn't. Unfortunately, like other cancers such as colon cancer, the first symptom is NO SYMPTOM. That is why screening is so essential. Yet, there are other signs to look out for.

Warning Signs:

Lump, hard knot in the breast.
A thickening in any part of the breast.
Nipple discharge that cannot be explained.
Painful itch within the breast.
Itchy, scaly or a sore nipple.
Swelling, warmth, redness or darkening that does not go away.
Inverted nipple or an indention in other parts of the breast.
New pain in one spot that persists.
Dimpling of the skin.
A change in the size of one breast compared to the other.

How to do Breast Self-Examination (BSE):

It should be done monthly and whenever you sense something isn't normal. You should check your breast, the chest area above and below your collarbone and your armpit.

1) In the shower, with soapy hands, raise you left arm and with your right hand and the pads of your fingers firmly touch every part of your left breast. Feel for lumps and thickening in the breast. Do the same with the other side
2) In a mirror raise your arms and look at both your breasts. Look for any changes in contour or shape. Check for any nipple discharge or inversion of the nipple. Check your underarm.
3) While lying down rub vertically over your breasts. Again you are looking for any irregularity.

Get a Mammogram

The American Cancer Society standard recommendation is to start at 40 but plenty of young women die from breast cancer *so if you think anything is wrong, are high risk or just want a base line test done, go get it done.*

The 2009 Government Preventative Task Force recommendations have suggested that women start at age 50, that the "net benefit" of starting younger is not significant. My personal opinion is that this is sending the wrong message – as though you don't need to worry about it until age 50. Nothing could be further from the truth. In 2010 a study out of Umea, Sweden, showed women who get regular mammograms in their 40's have a 26% greater survival rate.

Have a Doctor Examine You With Clinical Breast Examination (CBE)

This should happen during your yearly Ob-Gyn appointment. A physician should be more experienced with knowing what feels suspicious.

Monitor Your Body With Tests

If you are high risk or have any suspicion that something may be going on in your breast get tested even if you are young. Otherwise the ACS says you should have a baseline mammogram at 40 and one every year thereafter. Most breast cancers show up in women over 50 but they are more aggressive in younger women so to dismiss this because you are young is a mistake.

Eat Better and Supplement Your Diet

It just makes common sense that if you eat better – vegetables and fruits, good quality protein and plenty of clean drinking water – it will help support your body and immune system. Food is your fuel and a good multivitamin to cover your bases in the event you aren't getting all the vitamins especially vitamin D (in liquid or pill form) and minerals you need is a good idea. Along with good nutrition, flax seed and fish oil are also recommended by many dieticians.

No or Less Alcohol

Alcohol converts to sugar in the body. Tumors like sugar. Cutting down on sugar is smart. In addition, alcohol is hard on the liver and your liver is already working overtime to process the kinds of foods we already put into our system – a variety the human body has never before consumed, not to mention any medication you may be taking. The liver is the filtering system. The less you tax it the better.

Regular Exercise

Even walking is good. I find that I only *like* exercise when I do it often, otherwise it feels too hard. As we age increasing blood flow and strength training is important for our well-being and our bones.

Get Enough Sleep

Take your sleep seriously. Sleep is very restorative and a time of deep healing. While seemingly at rest your body continues to perform the necessary functions of breathing, digestion, brain function, swallowing, etc., which are all essential to your staying alive. Your body is also resetting, recharging and healing that which needs healing or at least it is trying to. Night pain is often a sign of inflammation somewhere in the body.

This is my sleep theory. It isn't scientific but it does come from personal experience. *Breast cancer woke me up in the middle of the night.* It woke me out of a deep sleep when my body was at rest. The attention of my energy zeroed in on my breast. I felt an activity in my chest that was startling enough to wake me up. Without this my breast cancer could have gone undetected for many years as there was no lump initially.

This is to say that what happens in your sleep matters. And desperate for sleep, a lot of Americans take sleep medicine. They attribute their dysfunctional sleep on stress and trick the body into sleep so as not to be disturbed. But perhaps your body is trying to tell you something and drugging it is only masking the symptoms. You may be turning off the very alarm you need to heed. Yes, there may be times when sleeping products are necessary – jetlag, after surgery when the pain of healing is keeping you awake, but I would suggest to you that over medicating your sleep is not letting your body speak to you. In this "go full speed ahead" American culture sleep gets a bad rap. "Lazy," "not ambitious," "what's wrong with him or her?" You wouldn't say that about someone who needs to eat food or drink water.

Yes, there are times when excessive sleeping is a dysfunction but I would argue that sleep is a much underrated health necessity. Everyone is different and some people don't require as much sleep but it is important to get what you need especially when your body is healing. There is a link between sleep and healing and not just when you are sick. Our functioning body is always trying to heal itself. Look at any child's scraped knee after a week of healing and you can't doubt the miracle of the body's ability to heal itself. An important concept to hold on to whether you are ill with cancer or not is this: *your body is naturally programmed to be well.*

Everyone needs sleep. You die without it. Protect it and know that its mysteries are not fully discovered. It may prove that your body is more aware of its condition while it sleeps than while it is awake. It could very well be that interrupted sleep is warning you your body needs help. Sleep, in my opinion, is like our internal mother. It gives us life, heals our cuts and nurtures us. If you numb it rather than pay it the respect it deserves and listen to the message it is trying to send you, you may be putting yourself in jeopardy. Listen while you sleep.

CAN BREAST CANCER BE PREVENTED?

No. Current modern medicine has no known way of preventing breast cancer. However, there are various behaviors and procedures (some drastic, some not) that have been shown to reduce the risk.

Nutrition

It would be common sense that good nutrition affects your overall health but again there are no clear studies that good nutrition prevents breast cancer. What is generally recommended is real colorful food (not processed), fish oil, flaxseed, fruits and vegetables, lean meat and a general low-calorie diet. Hormone-free food if possible. Take a multivitamin and ask your doctor's advice about additional supplements like vitamin D and calcium.

No Alcohol

There is a link between alcohol use and cancer.

No Smoking

Exercise

Limit Your Chemical Exposure Regarding Cleaning Supplies, Gardening and Cosmetics, including Deodorant.

Be Aware of Your Toxic Environmental Exposure and Limit It When Possible.

Prophylactic Mastectomy

This drastic procedure can't eliminate the chance of getting breast cancer completely but certainly greatly diminishes the risk.

AM I AT HIGER RISK THAN THE GENERAL POPULATION?

Trying to determine your risk for various diseases may be worthwhile but it may come with the need for behavior modification. Risk stratification does not mean you will get the disease but for some it is better to know where they are on the bell curve. It may make you more vigilant in monitoring your health especially around certain behaviors.

Age

As a woman gets older her chances of breast cancer increase. Most breast cancers in women are found after 50. However, being young does not make you risk free.

Prior History of Breast Cancer

A personal history of breast cancer automatically puts you at higher risk of getting the disease again.

Family History

Family history of breast cancer increases your risk. This includes your father's side of the family.

Obesity and Inactivity

Being overweight and inactive are thought to be risk factors.

Genetics

Inherited genetic mutations show up in BRCA 1 and BRCA 2 genes. Women who have these gene mutations have an 87% increased chance of developing breast cancer in their lifetimes.

Not Having Children or Having a First Child after 30

Not breast feeding, which "matures" the breast, increases risk.

Alcohol

Alcohol use has been shown to increase risk.

Ethnicity

There are two ethnic backgrounds which, according to the statistics, confer a higher risk for breast cancer than that of the general population: African American women and Ashkenazi Jews. Women in these groups tend to die younger and in higher numbers.

In the African American population there is both less education about the importance of early detection and less availability of actual screening which means women are also less likely to have the cancer detected in the early stages when it is most treatable. And in addition, African Americans also have a higher incidence of the aggressive triple negative type of breast cancer. Triple negative means that you are both ER (estrogen) and PR (progesterone) negative and you are also Her/2neu negative. Your treatment options are limited because common hormone therapy is not appropriate. As mentioned earlier, surgery and/or chemotherapy is the standard treatment for a triple negative diagnosis.

And, for unknown reasons, Ashkenazi Jewish people (women and men), have so far been determined to have the highest incidences of BRCA mutations. The BRCA mutation (gene variant) is linked to cell growth. You can inherit this gene mutation from *your mother or your father* which is sometimes overlooked as doctors concentrate on the maternal side of the family. And there seems to be no set time at which the cancer may develop, even among siblings. The gene information is available for a fee but the burden of the information is a heavy one; once you know your lifetime risk your choices become more obvious. Genetic counseling is highly advised. The site www.FORCE (Facing Our Risk of Cancer Empowerment) is dedicated to BRCA positive people.

TIP: It is important that doctors are aware of your Jewish heritage as they evaluate you. One woman I knew was not advised to have her BRCA status checked since she had an Italian last name – *it was her married name.* She was Jewish and in fact BRCA positive.

WHAT IF YOU ARE HIGH RISK?

Prophylactic Mastectomy

Some women who are at high risk choose prophylactic mastectomy. They have their breasts removed without any indication of having breast cancer or they ask to remove a healthy breast when it has been determined the other one has breast cancer. Women who have been diagnosed with the BRCA 1 and BRCA 2 gene mutations or women with a strong family history of breast cancer sometimes decide they would rather minimize their risk with this pro-active procedure. This, of course, is a huge decision and not for everyone but right for some. While even prophylactic mastectomy cannot guarantee you will never get breast cancer, as surgeons can't be certain they removed every last speck of breast tissue, it does greatly reduce your risk.

Tamoxifen

Tamoxifen is a drug that blocks estrogen. If you are at risk for cancer that is estrogen or progesterone positive (which means it is sensitive to the hormones estrogen and progesterone – not all breast cancers are) then tamoxifen might be prescribed. Tamoxifen is sometimes suggested for pre-menopausal high-risk women. The protocol has been to take the drug everyday for five years. It does have side effects and is not appropriate for all breast cancer patients. Again, only you and your doctor can decide if this is right for you. With any drug you want to assess the risk/benefit. For example if you have Stage 1 breast cancer (the tumor is less than 2 cm. and you are node negative) the chances of your surviving 5 years is 80% with surgery. Your chances only improve by another 5% if you take tamoxifen. Some studies have indicated tamoxifen substantially reduces the chances of your having breast cancer in your other breast.

BE YOUR OWN ADVOCATE

The most effective action I have taken for myself is being *an empowered patient.* The days of doctors being "nudges" have gone the way of the milkman. No one comes to your door delivering health care. You have to seek it out.

We were not taught in the 50s, 60s and 70s that health care

was completely our responsibility. There was still a partnership between doctor and patient that existed outside the doctor's office and hospital. I have been lucky to have a gentleman general practitioner, Dr. Paul Rudnick, who will still write a personal note to let you know the results of your tests but that personal touch is unusual, and for the most part there is no coddling in today's health care system.

I remember being a little girl and our family physician, Dr. Richard (Dick) Ziegler, would call the house. He would speak to my mother but by the time the conversation was done he had discussed everyone in the family and who needed what shot or medicine. And then, on the soccer field, as my brothers played with his kids you would hear him say to my mom, "Pat, call the office, come see me." He cared, he followed up. We were his patients and we were his friends. Yes, he even visited our house a few times when someone was really sick, my brother with mono, my dad with kidney stones. You always felt he was invested in our well-being.

Now doctors don't overstep the boundary. They are slammed for time, overwhelmed with information and administration requirements and concerned about malpractice. Rarely if ever do they hold your hand; only a few of them do and only if the world is crumbling. They are victims of the system too. And we could discuss ad infinitum how we got here and what should change but the real point I am trying to make is that the system is different than we were raised to believe (if you are over 40). The importance of this is critical

Unfortunately, "No news is good news" isn't fail-safe when it comes to breast cancer. Just because you feel good doesn't mean you are good. Cancer often doesn't hurt until it has already done some major damage.

11

New Science and Reconstruction Techniques

About 20% of the genetic information found in your nose does not match anything ever seen before.

–Nathan Wolfe

GENES, DO THEY ANSWER ALL THE QUESTIONS?

With the study of the Human Genome Project genes have become a yardstick to measure risk. This sensitive information contained in your genes may indicate your proclivity for being struck with diseases like cancer, heart disease, diabetes and Alzheimer's. Genes can't determine certitude; they can only imply greater risk. This information, while exciting in terms of perhaps heading off disease, can lead to a whole host of psychological and logistical questions. *The dilemma is if it isn't absolute certainty that the test is offering, how do you weigh the risk and what do you do with the information?*

The medical community doesn't yet know the complete answer when it comes to genes and breast cancer. There are at least two gene alterations that have been discovered with a link to breast cancer, BRCA 1 and BRCA 2. However, just because you have these gene mutations does not mean you will get breast cancer and on the flip side just because you don't have these gene mutations does not make you immune from breast cancer (your chances would revert to the norm – 1 in 8).

Yet the statistics are impactful if you have BRCA positive status. According to the American Cancer Society if you have these gene mutations you have approximately an 87% chance of getting breast cancer in your lifetime. However, if you have other invasive procedures, such as having your ovaries removed, your risk does go down. If you are BRCA positive the American Cancer Society suggests you have annual breast MRIs along with mammograms.

In 2012 we are on the cusp of the exciting area of "personalized medicine." Hope is that more targeted treatments will be tailored to the specific tumor markers of the disease. The emphasis will be to treat the pathology of the disease rather than just treating the body part.

Interventions based on a genetic likelihood have layers of complexity. As I mentioned, if you test positive for the gene mutations you have an 87% risk that you will get breast cancer in your lifetime. Currently there is no way to predict when it might happen from your genes. However, there are women whose parents have the gene alteration, they don't and yet they still get breast cancer. And while these gene mutations are linked to the disease the entire story of genes and breast cancer is still untold. There may be other gene mutations yet to be discovered that are more conclusive. Remember, the experts do not know what causes the disease. In cervical cancer, it has been determined that a virus can cause the disease. As a result of this discovery there is a vaccination for cervical cancer. This has not been ruled in or out for breast cancer. There is no vaccination for breast cancer nor do they know if a vaccine would be effective.

What is fueling this brave new world is not only the excitement of scientific breakthroughs but also a business model that shows real profit and growth. And where the business model is this lucrative and personally invasive, real checks and balances need to be in place. Issues of privacy and discrimination related to insurance, housing, employment, immigration, etc., have yet to be sorted out. So while it may be great news for women wanting answers related to their genes, the far-reaching implications of others knowing your "gene identity" have not been fully evaluated or regulated.

There is no governmental body, including the FDA, overseeing genetic testing. At present there are companies like Navigenics and Myraid that specialize in determining probability of disease with respect to your genes but that kind of information comes with a multitude of implications. The passing of GINA (federal legislation that protects consumers from insurance discrimination due to genetic testing) is an important milestone but concerns remain in the area of patient privacy when it comes to gene testing and they have not been completely addressed.

Over-the-counter testing kits are currently available to test for all kinds of predispositions based on your genes. Once again "the business" of medicine is ahead of the ethics and potential social impact.

WHAT IS GENETIC TESTING?

Genetic testing can provide a road map of your genetic make up. Two gene mutations, BRCA1 and BRCA 2, have been closely associated with inherited breast cancer and a more recent gene mutation, ARID1A, linked to ovarian cancer, has also been implicated as playing a role in breast cancer.

We all have these genes. It is the mutation, which damages the DNA, that puts you at risk. The normal function of BRCA and ARID1A genes is to act as tumor suppressants, in other words, when not damaged, these genes stop tumors. When mutated or damaged they allow DNA to be "mis-read" and "turned on." A blood test can determine if genes have mutated.

SHOULD I BE TESTED FOR BRCA1 and BRCA 2 GENE MUTATIONS?

This is a very personal decision as the results may leave you with more questions than answers. While as said before the risk for lifetime breast cancer is high if you have the mutation – 87% – it still cannot absolutely predict when or if you will develop breast cancer. So if you decide to be tested in order to "know," then you need to be prepared to deal with the information. It is important you see a genetic counselor *before* you submit to the test, for once you know the outcome of the test you may be tormented by the decision-making.

WHERE IS THE TEST DONE?

Myraid Labs in Salt Lake City holds the patent on the test and is the only place in the U.S. in 2011 where BRCA testing is done. Myraid first sends a package to your doctor and then you get your blood test done by your doctor or at a lab.

HOW MUCH DOES IT COST?

As of January 2012 it costs $3,120 for the BRCA test. This is for the comprehensive test. Note: once again everything but the cost was posted on the Myraid website. The company will tell you the cost when you ask.

WILL MY INSURANCE PAY FOR IT?

If you fall into certain high risk categories the test will be covered by insurance but you have to pay your co-pay and of course meet your deductible first. They use the date of the blood test for insurance purposes. This is important if you haven't met your deductible for the year.

WHAT ARE THE STATISTICS FOR BRCA 1?

According to Myraid the BRCA1 mutation means an up to 87% risk of breast cancer and 44% risk of ovarian cancer by age 70. A fifty percent chance of getting it before the age of 50.

WHAT ARE THE STATISTICS FOR BRCA 2?

According to Myraid the BRCA2 mutation means an up to 87% risk of breast cancer. And there is a slightly higher risk of male breast cancer – 6% more.

WHAT IS THE PROTOCOL WHEN YOU TEST POSITIVE FOR THESE GENE MUTATIONS?

The fact is the test is only a little over a decade old. This is definitely a case where the science is ahead of the studies for proven recommendations. That said, the current statistics would encourage someone to address this actively but the ball is in the patient's court given there is no actual disease present. Being pro-active when the chances of getting a disease are not certain, but very high, can be one of the most difficult decisions to make especially when this information comes at a very young age.

DOES HAVING PROPHYLACTIC MASTECTOMIES SECURE MY CHANCES OF NOT GETTING BREAST CANCER?

No, not absolutely. However, this is a common medical recommendation for women with the BRCA 1 or BRCA 2 mutation. Double mastectomy will by far greatly reduce your chances of getting breast cancer but even women who have had a bilateral mastectomy still have developed breast cancer as they can never be sure all the breast cancer tissue was removed. And of course this isn't an insignificant surgery.

Note: The idea that you would have both breasts removed often comes up when you are discussing any mastectomy – especially if you have already been diagnosed with the disease. Do you want to remove both breasts and reduce your chances of a new cancer in the other breast? Some women opt for this alternative. Again, this is what makes breast cancer complicated. There always seem to be options around the treatment and they often fall into the category of the lesser of two hard choices.

SHOULD I HAVE MY OVARIES REMOVED (OOPHORECTOMY)?

The chances of ovarian cancer increase with these mutations by up to 44% over your lifetime.

DECIDING ON PROPHYLATIC MASTECTOMY

The decision to have a prophylactic mastectomy is a daunting one for most women. In the face of no obvious disease, taking such a pro active step takes a lot of courage and thought. One woman I know made this decision primarily for her children. For eight years she lived with the knowledge that she was BRCA positive and her sister had breast cancer. She found the threat of the disease made her less attached and that caused her not to live as fully as she wanted, always waiting for the other shoe to drop and to be yanked off the stage so to speak. "I was living with a dark cloud over my life. I want to be free of it." She was another reminder that this genetic information, while valuable, comes at great cost and tremendous pressure to fix it. And sometimes the "fix" does not always turn out as you hoped as all surgery has trade-offs. Again, it is often the lesser of two bad choices.

Recently I met another woman that had the information for years and put off the procedure, even though her mother died from breast cancer. She is now dealing with the disease and in addition to guilt and sadness that she didn't act earlier when she had a chance to head it off. But again it is a personal and heart-wrenching choice.

WHAT IF MY BREASTS HAVE BEEN AUGMENTED WITH IMPLANTS?

With our cultural obsession with breasts, particularly large ones, implants, previously popular primarily in the entertainment and sex industries, have now become commonplace. But they should come with a warning – *buyer beware*. Implants are not without consequences when it comes to breast cancer although you wouldn't know it given the popular media coverage.

As I have watched the plastic surgery shows currently on television, I have yet to hear the topic of breast cancer come up in the consultations between doctors and their patients when they discuss augmentation. If you were to get your information solely from these shows you would think that there was no impact whatsoever.

There are in fact unintended consequences of augmentation when it comes to breast cancer. Implant safety is of course a concern. While implants have been approved for use, the safety and reliability of saline and silicone implants is still being studied. In addition, the ability to detect breast cancer and diagnose it properly if an implant is in place is at issue.

According to the book *Breast Cancer: from the M.D. Anderson's Cancer Care Series*, "Mammographic screening is more difficult in patients who have had previous breast augmentation, especially if the implant was placed in-retro glandular rather than sub-muscular position." And, "once an abnormality is detected in the woman with breast implants, the diagnostic approach needs to be carefully selected to avoid injury to the implant. And there is even the possibility that the lymphatic route is altered as a result of the implantation, making the option of a sentinel node biopsy not as reliable if breast cancer is diagnosed. This problem reflects a disruption of lymphatics during implant placement."

These are all issues that should be discussed not only with your plastic surgeon but with a breast cancer expert prior to implantation. I believe every women considering augmentation should be counseled by a breast cancer expert first in order to fully assess her individual risk and the potential long term impact.

There also seems to be a trend where women over 40 who have had their children and want to restore the look of their bodies to pre-pregnancy are more and more opting for augmentation. This coincides with the time when their breast cancer risk increases due to age and yet in many cases they are not being made aware of the added complexities of screening or are choosing to ignore them.

With early detection as our best offensive move against breast cancer, it is important for any woman considering implants to at least be made aware of the potential difficulties in early detection and possible complications if breast cancer were to present itself.

NEW BREAST RECONSTRUCTION OPTIONS

If I had to face reconstruction now, in 2012, I would consider a new method that results in a more natural look. Dr. Karl H. Breuing, a plastic surgeon who specializes in breast reconstruction, is doing a cutting-edge procedure using an acellular dermal matrix, like AlloDerm® or Strattice, that is offering superior results.

When it comes to reconstruction, not all options are always reviewed by either patient or surgeon and what is offered or discussed frequently depends on the training and expertise of the doctor you are consulting. As Dr. Breuing, formerly of Brigham & Women's Hospital in Boston, now visiting professor in Hannover, Germany, says "Without all the information, women are not fully empowered and are often forced to make a decision without really understanding the consequences of their choices. The options don't have to be as rigid as they are often presented. They should be tailored to a woman's individual needs."

Most women tend to make a decision regarding reconstruction in the first weeks of diagnosis but he advises, "There is no need to rush to a decision." This haste prevents the patient from being able to consider all the options or to do proper research. In his opinion, patients should not just look at photos, but if possible should meet with other patients and discuss their overall experiences. In his practice, he suggests women interview several of his patients who have had different types of reconstructions and/or other individuals who have been treated for breast cancer before making a decision. It is only after talking with other patients about the process, learning about the pros and cons of their experience and seeing the final outcome that you can make a fully informed decision.

In a typical implant reconstruction, an expander is almost always placed first to establish a pocket into which a final implant (silicone or saline) would be inserted. In cases where women either had previous radiation or will need to have radiation as part of their therapy, most plastic surgeons are reluctant to use implants as radiation can slow the healing process and can change the skin's elasticity over time. This in turn increases the chance of developing unpredictable scar formations around the implant, so-called capsular contractures. The body tends to create "capsules" or coats around any foreign body or implant and so any implant will also result in formation of a capsule. Ideally it remains smooth and has no visible effect, but if this capsule starts to harden and contract significantly, the result can be painful and rather unsightly. The amount of capsular contracture can be graded from 1 to 4. Grade 4 means it is painful and looks like the breast is being squeezed against the body. Capsular contracture is something every patient and surgeon wants to avoid. That is why until recently plastic surgeons have been reluctant to use implants when the skin has been irradiated as you can never reliably predict how the tissue will behave.

Fortunately for those who prefer not to have a TRAM or other muscle/fat based flaps, and for whom an implant reconstruction is really the best option, there is a groundbreaking procedure to consider. Based on careful review of the literature and clinical studies regarding the use of biomaterials in plastic surgery, Dr. Breuing's pioneering technique involves the use of an "acellular dermal matrix" (either AlloDerm® or Strattice™) as a sling to hold the implant in place. With this technique more natural skin is preserved at the time of the mastectomy, often making an expander unnecessary and allowing for immediate placement of the actual implant in one procedure. That then also obviates the need for the frequently painful repeated expansion process. Even if for various reasons an expander does need to be placed initially (due to insufficient native skin envelope for instance), using this acellular dermal matrix still makes the expansion process less uncomfortable and allows for more rapid expansion to the desired size. This strap or hammock technique allows for more natural movement of the implant reconstructed breast. The matrix, made from cadaver or pig skin, is placed over the full-size implant or expander and essentially cradles it. As he describes it, "Biomechanically the matrix has the right structure, so the body doesn't seem to mind its presence and in fact starts to populate it with its own cells." This matrix material is tried and proven and has been used for years for support or reconstruction in other parts of the body such as hernia repairs, bladder reconstructions, rhinoplasties (noses) and even as coverage for burn wounds.

Dr. Breuing explains, "What is wonderful about this technique is we can now offer patients a more natural result with one surgery or with a much shorter expansion process and diminish the chances of capsular contracture. While great results can be achieved with autologous (using one's own tissue) reconstruction, I see a lot of young women who are BRCA positive and really struggle with the decision to have a prophylactic double mastectomy and having to sacrifice other parts of their body in order to reconstruct their breasts. Being able to offer them a simpler, yet very natural looking solution that is less invasive and has fewer complications is very rewarding and often helps them to make such a major decision. Or for women who will need radiation therapy in the course of their treatment and thus have a higher risk of developing capsular contracture but who do not want to delay their reconstruction. In these situations, this technique provides a very good alternative."

He cautions that any one-sided reconstruction is never going to be exactly symmetrical and that the best way to get symmetry, if that is very important to you, is to reconstruct both sides at the same time. That said, it is understandable many women want to hold on to their native breasts as long as possible.

In his view reconstruction needs to be more of a "personally unique process. You are an individual and your needs are individual. We, the physicians, are there to help and fortunately, now there are tools available that allow us to tailor therapy to those needs."

Dr. Karl H. Breuing with a handful of other surgeons has spearheaded this technique of using acellular dermal matrices in breast and hernia surgery. To date these procedures are being offered throughout the U.S. and now increasingly also in Europe.

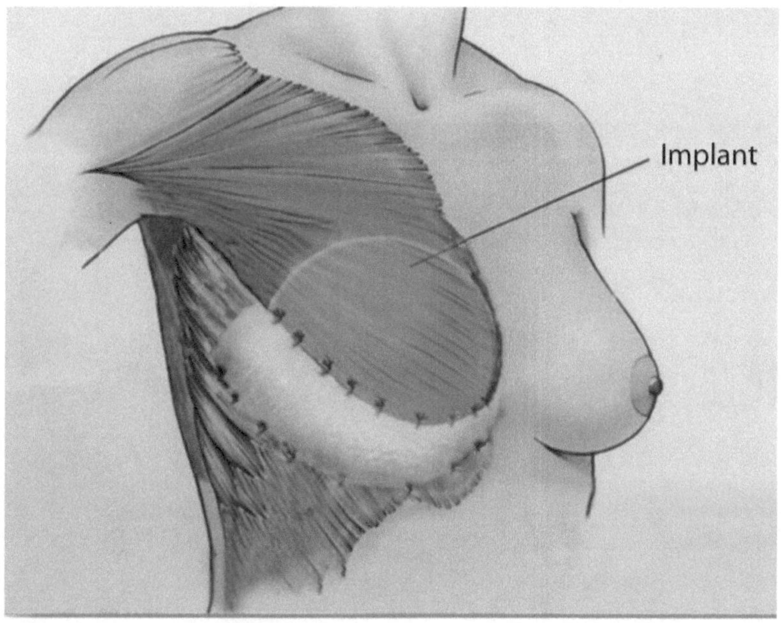

Reconstruction of a breast post mastectomy with AlloDerm®.

STEM CELL-ASSISTED LIPOTRANSFER

Another cutting-edge technique for reconstruction now available in the U.S. is a procedure that was developed in Japan by Dr. Kotaro Yoshimura which utilizes autologous adipose-derived adult stem cells in conjunction with liposuction. This procedure is now available through Dr. Joel Arnowitz's Outpatient Surgical Stem Cell Laboratory at St John's Medical Center in Santa Monica. This is in the very early stages of use and development but basically it uses the liposuction technique to harvest fat which includes stromal vascular faction containing stem-cells which are then isolated. The stem cell rich fat (ASC-rich fat) is then implanted into the patient and the fat acts as a scaffold for the growth. This enriched transplanted fat with stem cells increases the survival of the fat grafts.

12

Where is God?

I want to know the mind of God. The rest are details.

–Albert Einstein

Serious illness accelerates change in us and change, in the human experience, is most often accompanied by resistance. Breast cancer brings hyper-change. However, once some of the resistance to the reality of the diagnosis turns to acceptance, defenses may deconstruct. A shift in consciousness, even temporarily, is not uncommon. For many, their faith in God and church organizations offers safe haven. It can be a way to shift the burden. "I am not in control. God is." For others, they ask, "Where is God? If he was a loving and powerful being he would make this go away. Or he wouldn't have allowed this to begin with, would he?"

Clearly, breast cancer, like any serious set-back, can trigger you to question your core beliefs. It certainly alters our experience. Without breast cancer we would have had one experience, with it quite another. It is natural to ask the question, "Why me?"

When a doctor tells you that you have cancer it is not unusual to ask, "Will I die?" An odd question really because, of course, we all die. What we really want answered is, "Will I die of breast cancer, and when, and how, and will I be in pain, and will I be alone, and will I be able to get treatment?" And the list goes on. All these questions underline the fear and the uncertainty.

The cancer seems to, at every turn, strip you of so much, things we perhaps always took for granted – our health, our hair, our breasts, our eyelashes, our peace of mind, often our fertility and the possibility of our future. It is as though it is making a promise to take your body, your time and your special dreams and you want it to break its promise.

Holding on to the concept that the body, in its natural state, is on a path of healing can be like grabbing at the wind. But remember the scrape of your knee that healed in a week when you were a kid and know that your body is always making its best effort to renew and rejuvenate.

Fear of pain and fear of death. It is the fear which is heart-stopping and it is the fear which is driving much of the conversation and anxiety. Contemplating one's mortality is not usually what a human being does unless there is a threat to it. While we are healthy a false sense of immortality rules us. Serious illness makes you ask how much time you have left on earth and what will make for quality time. Of course every human faces a finite amount of time in this physical world – nothing new there – but we generally don't actively come to terms with this until we are elderly or we are given what appears to us to be a premature wake-up call.

Eckhart Tolle in his book *A New Earth* talks about the "inner purpose" and "outer purpose." That there needs to be a stripping away in order for us, if we are ready, to find our outer purpose. A breast cancer diagnosis can act as a potent stripper. There are, however, easier ways to get there, I assure you.

For many women going through their treatment a common refrain is "one day at a time." I remember in the thick of it when I had to reduce this down to "one minute at a time." This kind of crisis can make you become present to the moment, present to the day, present to the simple things that perhaps before you neglected to notice. You stop doing so much because you must and you are forced to just be, and in the being you realize you, the way you always defined you, perhaps isn't so accurate. That you aren't the car-pooler, the secretary, the dinner maker, the house cleaner, the executive, the real estate agent or the person who owns the house. Yes that is what you do, and maybe what you own but, that is not who you are. Because when you stop doing and owning you are still *being*. And it is in the being, the now, we can find out who we really are and we get to know others. Perhaps we recognize their spirit more fully because now we know what essence really looks like.

The night of my mastectomy, when I was having an allergic reaction to latex and fighting for air, my brother Fred sat in the corner of the hospital room from 4 to 11 P.M. I would wake occasionally but I had been given so much Benadryl that I was groggy and in and out of sleep. We didn't talk much but whenever I opened my eyes he was there. What I remember was not "his doctoring" but "his being" which was so powerful.

Over the next few months the world slowed for me or I should say I slowed in the world. I was only about being as I could do very little. So I would just sit and talk to friends and family and they would just sit and talk to me. I was driven to things rather than driving. I was a passenger, accepting the attention and care of others. It allowed a space for intimacy, friendship and companionship that is often obliterated by the constant doing of things. This is the space for the transformative part of cancer I believe. It forces you to slow down to just *be*.

While you may feel a shift within you, the day-to-day pressures of a diagnosis and your life may still be overwhelming. This is of course why many recommend support groups or seek out mental health professionals. If you've never had a therapist you may find having one now especially helpful. It is important to have friends and family you can rely on but you may need more structure or less judgment. The point is, you get to decide what gives you support and comfort.

TIP: When it comes to your mental health assess what works for you. Support groups may offer comfort for some but others find them depressing, not able to process the concerns of others while they are dealing with so much in their own lives. Many have found solace in their faith and church. Some need more time with people, some need more time alone. Often a personal therapist is necessary. Talking to a professional – not family or friend –where you can express without filter what is going on with you can be freeing. The point being, what is supportive for you may not be standard behavior. Give yourself permission to try what you think may work for you and to let go of it if it isn't working – there is no "should."

A cancer diagnosis can make you reflect on your religious beliefs. I was raised Catholic but these days I have a broader view. Surviving breast cancer is all about healing and this part of my story is about spiritual healing.

April 2006. One of my godchildren (I have five), is going to have her bat mitzvah in Israel. This trip was significant in many ways but there is one part that I would like to relay here for anyone reading this in the hope it may offer some comfort.

I have always wanted to go to Israel. I spent a junior year of college abroad in England and traveled all over Europe but never made it to the Middle East. Finally, I was getting to the place I had heard so much about. As I said, I was raised Catholic and although I no longer go to church regularly, I do believe in God and in an intelligent, benevolent power that continually offers us a positive path to enlightenment and love. I feel it is our choice to live there or not. I have also had many Jewish boyfriends and have been to more Passovers than the typical Catholic girl so the refrain "next year Jerusalem" sounds very familiar to me.

When the plane landed in Tel Aviv I actually had tears in my eyes. Another dream realized. I've always considered seeing the globe one of the real privileges of life. It also happened to be an especially holy time with Easter, Passover and Mohammed's birthday all happening that week. We stayed in Jerusalem but spent the week touring and visited Masada, the West Bank, up to the Lebanon border and Tel Aviv. It was prior to the last Lebanon war and the country felt peaceful although seeing soldiers with machine guns was not uncommon.

On Easter Saturday, the day after Good Friday and before Easter Sunday, I told my friends that I wanted to walk around the old city of Jerusalem. We had visited it and gone to the Western Wall and the market, but I felt I hadn't explored any of the Christian sights and I wanted to do some of that before I left the next day. My friend and her cousin decided to come with me.

As the three of us entered the Old City we noticed a man sitting on a rock. He asked us, "Do you know where you are going? Do you need help?" Now that I reflect on those questions it makes me wonder, "Is this what a guardian angel would say?" We didn't have a map or much time, so a guide would be helpful. He said he was Armenian but we later found out he was Palestinian. We explained to him we wanted to see some of the Christian sights and he offered to take us around.

Down a narrow path and through a stone doorway, we went into the room where The Last Supper took place. Ten young Asian women were harmoniously chanting and praying on the steps, a Jewish man holding a baby was davening and praying in the corner facing west. The whole room was made of stone but it was warm with every surface worn and smooth from so many curious hands. From there we went to the tomb of King David. We walked past the remains of the Roman marketplace to the Church of the Holy Sepulchre. It is here that a slab of stone, the Stone of Unction, which held the body of Jesus prior to burial, rests. A beautiful ancient mosaic is above it depicting the scene.

My friend wanted me and her cousin to visit the tomb of Jesus because when she was there once before, she had experienced the energy of the room and found it to be very powerful. Her cousin, a beautiful 26-year-old-girl, had been ill also and she felt the two of us needed healing. The church was crowded with tourists and followers, especially during this holy week. In Hebrew, she asked the Greek Orthodox priests who ran this part of the church to let us go in and pray. Our Palestinian tour guide took over and negotiated. The Greek Orthodox priest looked at both of us curiously – one of us Brazilian and one American, we both look like the picture of health. My friend told him again in Hebrew, "We were not well. We needed healing." He studied us again, a bit dubiously but I suppose truth is obvious because he said yes, but he would only let the two of us in. The international negotiations were concluded and successful.

The Chapel of the Angel is like a little house inside the church. It has an anteroom you step inside before entering the cave-like area where the tomb is located. We waited in the anteroom with a couple of priests. All my years of Catholic training seemed to flood my mind. How many "Our Fathers" had I prayed as a little kid? What would my mother, someone who fully embraced the church, think of my being here? Sense of smell is powerful and the smell of incense transported me back to New Jersey and St. Gregory's Church, where I made my first communion and where I practiced religion because I was forced to before I knew much about the history or tradition. For me, the energy inside this chapel was indeed overpowering.

To this day I am not completely sure what exactly I was feeling other than deep reverence but I don't underestimate it. A priest spoke and broke my daydream and asked us where we were from. I remember when I said, "Los Angeles," he responded smiling, "Hollywood?" I did think that was so funny – even at the tomb of Jesus they were fascinated with Hollywood. On reflection I think it was an effort for commonality and connection – his attempt to relate to me.

When it was our turn we had to duck through a small opening, about 4 feet high, to get to where the actual tomb was located. It is all made of stone – the tomb and the room so there is an impenetrable feeling that goes along with the space and yet I felt a high energy that accompanied the glow of the candlelight. Inside we both knelt by the worn Jerusalem stone. A simple silver bucket was there with white candles stuck in the sand. We each took a candle, lit them and prayed.

I thought about my parents, so long gone by now. I thought about the apparent fragility of my health. I thought about the life and goodness of Jesus – how did he always turn the other cheek, how did he face adversity with acceptance? I prayed for good health for me and for my friends and family. And then I remember asking in prayer, "Will I be okay?" Memories of hospital rooms flashed in my head. It was very emotional and in that moment I honestly was without reservation giving it up to God. "How is this going to turn out?" What happened next I have no explanation for, all I know it is what I experienced. A very clear and calm voice I have never heard before or since, said to me, "You are my daughter." It seemed like a voice from an eternal sound stage. The assurance of safety in those words was powerful and addressed every cell in my body. Even writing those words now brings me back to that moment and a feeling of peace. I left there thinking, no matter what, I am, *like all women*, a daughter of God and it is all going to be okay.

I believe that we are in our essence ancient and eternal. That, as Dr. Wayne Dyer often says, we are spiritual beings having a human experience. On earth we have suffering, much of it from resistance, but the suffering is real and should not be minimized. There is real physical pain, tragedy and torture and a lot of it appears to us unfair. What I know about a cancer diagnosis is it made me reflect and go deeper into my spirit. I feel the edge of physical life, like a cliff that drops off – sharp and distinctive. The fog has lifted and I sense the transition on the perceptible horizon.

I can't touch it but I now know it is there like a dream I will surely have. In the meantime to contain and transform the fear makes it easier to deal with the disease. That is why it is important to do so. And if faith can play a part then by all means allow it to be part of your experience.

Conventional religion may not be your answer. Search out whatever you find to be healing and comforting as it will be an individual expression of how you want to be. Yoga, meditation, walking in nature, playing with your pet, helping others, spending more time with friends, bike riding with your children or alone, painting or drawing or journaling. If these are healing things for you then they are not frivolous or a waste of time, but on the contrary, are essential to your well-being.

In late 2007 I prayed for God to "use me." Show me where I can serve. I didn't know exactly what would come up or when. Little things did but nothing as clearly as what came next.

In February 2008 I called my brother Fred to wish him happy birthday. He told me news that took my breath away. Amanda, my niece, had a tumor in her leg. When the diagnosis came back it was a pareosteal osteoscarcoma and we were all in shock. She needed to have a hip replacement and a femur resection at the age of 22.

There had been no warning. Typical of cancer she had not been in pain but felt a slight bulge of muscle on her one leg and luckily went to the doctors. She is 5'3" and weighed 110 pounds and in otherwise good health. The previous March I had taken her to the island of St. Martin as a graduation present from college and here we were a year later.

On March 10, 2008, I flew to Boston and on March 11 she had the surgery. I stayed in Boston with her for a month while she was in the hospital and for the start of her recovery. We are all hopeful that the low-grade quality of the tumor made surgery a successful treatment and she will have no more complications. Cancer had shown up again in our family and this time it seemed more unfair than ever.

There were so many times, as Amanda was recovering, I asked God, "Why?" At 22 she was in the first year of her first job at Boston Children's Hospital and her future so bright. I am still left wondering.

While this book is mostly about how to cope with and fight the disease, sometimes all the fight in the world does not make the disease relent. There are many who have understood the news of a cancer diagnosis and fought to the best of their capacity and know, regardless of their hard-fought battle, this isn't going to turn out as they had hoped. Sometimes all the faith and fight in the world doesn't make the cancer go away. They very well may lose their life due to breast cancer.

Cancer books, especially written by survivors, want to be the beacon of hope and therefore eschew discussing death, the potential elephant in the room. I assume this book will be read by many who will not die of breast cancer, but some will. And if you are reading this book with someone in mind, some of those people may die of breast cancer too. If that is the case for you, please say directly what you need to say to the people you need to say it to before it is too late. By the way, it is never too early to tell someone you love them and how much they mean to you, only too late. Don't be too late. Declaring our love and affection can be the most healing thing we will ever do. Expressing love, like fighting cancer, takes bravery.

There may be some who will read this book at the middle or even at the end of their fight. While a patient often experiences denial as a coping mechanism, family members and friends can be caught in the shelter of it too. And while it can have its usefulness and benefit, denial is often something the patient may come to terms with before family and friends. While it can be comforting to have people not give up hope, it can also create pressure on the patient that they are "letting you down." So compounding the sorrow around losing one's own life, you feel that you have disappointed those who love you by not continuing to fight. How sad that you should die without peace in spite of how valiantly you have endured because others may not be ready to let you go.

In 2010, at the age of 37, the actress Jennifer Lyon, lost her fight with breast cancer. Ironically, she had appeared on the show "Survivor." The quote that was attributed to her upon her death was, "I want them to know I fought the cancer." She didn't want to be viewed as giving up. I know of another example where a father desperate for his daughter to live, kept on pushing her to seek out new doctors and new treatments beyond the time when another doctor or drug was the answer. Acceptance, for some, does not come easily.

But I want to remind you, this is your path. That while others can be there for support, you are the one facing the disease with all its repercussions. So when it is clear that medicine, a new doctor, another treatment will not be able to save you or improve the quality of your life try to reframe their insistence on your fighting or continuing treatment as a "love life jacket" – one they need to wear in order to survive it. And then do what you feel is right for you.

Many say "this isn't fair." But fairness is not natural. Fairness springs from our humanity. Fairness, while laudable, does not run the universe nor is it a principle of the larger operating system, but a wonderful enhancement we as human beings have cultivated over time. Much of our sadness comes from our assumption that fairness is a law of nature and therefore we are stunned when cancer doesn't surrender to it. But nature is about survival not fairness. Children wouldn't lose their moms, husbands wouldn't lose their wives and women wouldn't lose their fight against breast cancer if fairness were part of the equation.

So you may still be left with the question "Where is God?" You may only find him in the small gestures, in nature, in the love you feel from others, and you may never get a satisfactory answer before this is over. You may have to rely on faith that there is a larger picture, one he or she created.

13

The Health Care Industry

I think this debate shows a fundamental lack of vision, a lack of confidence, a lack of understanding of what's possible.

– Dean Kamen, Inventor

For a good part of 2009 and 2010 health care reform dominated the political conversation and in 2010 the U.S. Congress passed legislation and President Obama signed into law Bill 3590, now in 2012 commonly known as the Affordable Care Act and "Obamacare."

While this was presented as a health care reform bill, it was really a bill that addressed health insurance issues more than the actual delivery of health care. And while most agree the health care system needed changes, it is wise to keep in mind that every action creates a reaction. Sweeping changes that do more harm (more bureaucracy, more expense, more complications, less health *care*, more lawsuits, less prevention, less monitoring) are not what we need. And given, the IRS was always tasked with the power and responsibility to enforce the "fine portion" of the law, the fact that the mandate was ultimately termed a "tax" by the Supreme Court and therefore constitutional, should not have been a surprise. If it stands, the full effect of all the provisions of this bill will be years in the making.

What Americans are spending on treatment of disease has skyrocketed. And I say "treatment of disease" because the health care dollar is spent, for the most part, on disease and not prevention or early detection. It is also spent on emergency services for the 47 million Americans uninsured for they have nowhere else to go. However, emergency rooms do not offer chemotherapy and other similar modalities and are not equipped to treat cancer, which leaves millions in a hospital room with the taxpayer footing the bill. It is also spent on expensive and wasteful defensive medicine due to the threat of lawsuits. And there is the simple fact that 5% of the patients are accounting for 50% of the costs because when you are very sick it is very expensive.

Without insurance you have a much greater chance of dying from cancer than with insurance. This is due in part to lack of good continuous overall care, health education and the fact those without insurance are less likely to have cancer and other serious illnesses detected early, when they are more treatable.

Even with insurance women under 50, who have previously been healthy, often have very little experience with the health care system. So not only are they dealing with a serious disease they are also learning about the health care system and its shortcomings, perhaps for the first time, and the learning curve is steep.

What I have tried to outline in this book is a way to help you manage the system as related to medical issues. To empower you to ask questions, negotiate and discuss your options with your physicians in order to receive the best care you are entitled to.

Assuming you are one of the lucky ones and at least have insurance, insurance bills and doctor bills can still make you feel like you are under constant attack. I have had surgical procedures under anesthesia and gotten an unexpected bill, not realizing the anesthesia portion wasn't part of the original surgery quote, a year and half later. The anesthesiologist's fee was not covered and never came up in the financial conversation I had with the surgeon. I did not see the anesthesiologist until the day of the surgery, which is typical. I certainly didn't ask him what his fee was dressed in my hospital gown. I had erroneously assumed the anesthetic was part of the surgery price. Doesn't it make sense that the cost of being sedated would be part of the surgery? It isn't like it is optional.

Or the time I chose to go with a surgeon not in my insurance system (in-network) to fix a prior botched reconstruction, fully expecting the insurance company would understand that I didn't have much of a choice, I needed her unique skills and special expertise. I assumed they would pay her a fair amount. The surgery was quoted in cash because she knew the insurance company would pay very little of her fee and she was right.

TIP: If you opt to have surgery ask your surgeon what the entire surgery will cost – including hospital stay and other medical costs. The anesthesiologist is often a separate cost and one that you should be aware of prior to surgery. Get the anesthesiologist's phone number prior to the surgery and ask about the fee.

TIP: If you choose a doctor or surgeon outside of your insurance company network, remember this could be an ongoing relationship and therefore not a onetime cost. If you need continuous care (from say, an oncologist) or perhaps a follow-up surgery (as I did) you will be faced with another bill your insurance company won't pay. This could very well end up being thousands of dollars and may impact how rigorously you look for someone who practices within your insurance plan (in-network).

Our health care system is a combination of public and private funding but it is regulated by the government. It is an all-licensed field (doctors, pharmacies, hospitals, drug companies, labs) and the licenses are granted by the government. You can't get a test, receive medicine, treatment or surgery without being part of the government-regulated system. While this allows for standards to protect the consumer it also has sheltered those that serve a captive audience and encouraged nothing less than gross abuse in terms of profit-making, especially by insurance and drug companies.

All one has to do is to look at the balance sheets of drug and insurance companies and then try to tell me they aren't capitalizing on an option-less, controlled and vulnerable public. In 2010 one drug company, Pfizer, made 67.8 billion dollars. Herceptin, one cancer-fighting drug, was over a 1 billion dollar business in 2009. A CEO of a health insurer made 200 million dollars in 2009.

But what choice do we as consumers really have? We are hostages to the system especially if you have had a serious illness. A new insurance company doesn't want to put you on its rolls and if they do the cost will be exorbitant to be sure. To what degree this will be addressed in the new legislation has yet to be actualized; while they have said you can't be denied insurance for pre-existing conditions the cost of that insurance has yet to be determined. If you cannot afford the premium the new rule is irrelevant. And to what degree the cost of the new law to the insurance companies will be passed on to all consumers has yet to be calculated but it will no doubt make it more expensive for everyone. Let's face it... when was the last time a cost went down?

Some Americans are choosing to go abroad for treatment to avoid such an expensive system. They (the doctors, the AMA, hospitals, FDA, drug companies, insurance companies and our government) have a lock on it. There is no domestic alternative. You have to pay their fees and abide by their rules. At the same time the costs have skyrocketed and there is no one to negotiate with, or they are in hiding, or so it seems.

I believe that they (the hospitals, the insurance and drug companies) like the lack of transparency. A non-transparent system is the system they have set up and it works to their benefit. If it didn't they would change it. They pay millions to lobbyists in order to gain the favor of politicians. Have you noticed insurance companies and drug companies don't broadcast their lobbying costs?

The health crisis we are in isn't just about people without insurance. The costs are so prohibitive that it is affecting those insured as well. And it is getting worse every year as the population increases and more and more people are not covered and costs have inflated. Simply put, people can no longer afford the premiums. Medical bills are the number one reason for bankruptcies in America.

Another issue is that your state health insurance, while possibly covering you in another state for an emergency or treatment if you have pre-approval, has not been transferable if you move to another state. As of 2011 you can not buy insurance across state lines. And even if there is a "converter plan" it is usually much more expensive with wait times. So what do you do if you have a pre-existing issue and need to move to another state? You may have to enter a high-risk pool but sometimes the high-risk pools that states have set up don't allow you to even join if you haven't established residency for 12 months (i.e. Kentucky Access). With the new Bill 3590 they are not allowed to deny you coverage if you have a pre-existing condition but again the cost of your premium has yet to be determined. The fact is the iceberg of good care at affordable prices has already melted away for most Americans.

The health care question is undoubtedly complicated but we can't continue on this path. Too many are uninsured and too many who are insured still can't pay for what they need. Everyone is likely to need care at some point and there is really no way of predicting, in every case, who will need expensive care. We need to honestly *ask and answer* the hard question, *who is going to pay for it? What does basic care include? Does the patient bear all the cost, any of the cost or some of the cost? What is the responsibility of an employer?*

The new Bill 3590 stipulates that employers with 50 or more employees must offer health insurance or pay a fine. Will the fines be less expensive than offering the health care?

Some say the government should pay as in a single payer system but we don't know what the unintended consequences would be. Would it mean long lines? Wait times? A decline in quality? Rationing? Would it encourage a private, cash side business that only the rich will be able to afford? Will health care go the way of the public school system? As the population ages and the technology and kind of medical procedures increase can we afford to pay for every treatment? Who decides what is necessary? The patient? The doctor? The insurance company? In Los Angeles and many other places, doctors are already setting up a system where patients must "join" in order to get the services of a certain doctor. Without paying a yearly fee to the doctor, the services of that doctor are no longer available to them.

And the argument that "if you like your current health care you can keep it" is a faulty one. Due to added government regulations and requirements the cost of your health care, if you are self-employed, may become prohibitive. I just checked on my policy and they told me they were "government mandated to add maternity" among other things to my policy. Benefits I will never use but will be added to the cost. There is no common sense.

Historically hospitals would set a fee for a procedure, drug or device and then the insurance company would negotiate the price they are willing to pay the hospital for that procedure, drug or device. The premise here is insurance companies pay a "discounted price" for the procedure because they are big customers and carry a lot of leverage with the hospitals. In other words, because the insurance companies have so many customers they have leverage over the hospitals – the providers of the care. The hospital and doctors in order to get the business went along with the reduced fees. This worked relatively fine for some time but things have changed drastically.

This worked as long as deductibles were low, doctors were in the system, co-pays were low, hospitals had a handle on waste, the population was younger, the amount of treatments available were smaller, litigation was less, people were insured and costs were under control.

All those elements have changed. Premiums have skyrocketed. Deductibles and co-pays aren't low anymore, many doctors have opted-out of the system due to low reimbursements from insurance companies and Medicare, hospitals do not have a handle on waste, the population is getting older with more people uninsured, the number of treatments and drug protocols available have increased dramatically as well as the costs, malpractice insurance has skyrocketed due to claims and the costs of treatment and drugs have increased. We are left with insurance companies making medical decisions because they impact their bottom line. This has resulted in some patients going abroad for their surgical needs and paying cash at reduced rates rather than the outrageous sums the same surgery or treatment requires in the States. Is going to India for your cancer treatment or hip replacement part of the American Dream? Do we really want to outsource our healthcare?

The government is already a dominant player in our health care system. Medicare (a federal program) and Medicaid (joint federal and state) are two mammoth government-funded entities. Together they make up 19% of the federal 2009 budget (676 billion dollars) without counting the state contribution. What is troubling for many is that these systems are infested with bureaucracy, unfairness, fraud and waste which I think is the basis for the fear behind "government run" health care. If the government can't run the systems they already have under their control efficiently why would we want them to take on more? And in their current form it is unsustainable, simply put, they are going broke.

Under the current system a Medicare patient (someone who is over 65, people under 65 with certain disabilities and people with kidney failure on dialysis) or a Medicaid patient (someone whose health insurance is covered by the government and whose eligibility is based mostly on financial resources of the individual) receives treatment and then the government reimburses the provider or servicer. The reimbursements have been declining over the years – an inverse relationship to the costs.

According to the AMA, in Massachusetts, at the current rate by 2013 Medicare reimbursements to physicians will be less than half of what they were in 1991. In some cases these reimbursements have been so low that doctors are opting out – the fees don't cover their expenses. They are losing money as they work and yet are still legally responsible for their patients. All the while medical malpractice rates, the cost of the operation and cost of running an office and business have gone up. We are essentially asking doctors to operate (sometimes in the middle of the night), take on all the liability and *lose* money. It makes no sense and it is an unsustainable model. In addition, the government has gotten more and more involved in the medical decisions around the actual surgery which, if not followed to the letter, impact if a doctor gets reimbursed at all. For example, the government dictates timelines for giving antibiotics around a surgery. If for some reason this is not followed exactly the doctor does not get reimbursed. Do we really want government making antibiotic care decisions?

Keep in mind if a hospital participates in Medicare (and most do) there is a 1986 federal law giving everyone the right to emergency care at that hospital regardless of your ability to pay. What the law essentially entitles you to in an emergency room is "stabilizing care" for a patient with a medical emergency. This means screening, emergency care and appropriate transfer once the patient has been stabilized. However, if it is not an emergency the hospital does not have to treat you. For any treatment you will be billed and who pays is between you and your insurance company or you and the hospital.

Insurance companies are regulated by the state in which they operate. This is one of the reasons buying insurance across state lines has been prohibited. The initial purpose of this was to insure, through state control, that the insurance companies would be solvent. Odd really as many states haven't been fiscally prudent themselves – they make a lame watchdog. But at this point regulations and cost of entry into the health insurance business make it near impossible for new competitors to enter the marketplace. Still, that is the way it works right now. So insurance companies set up different entities under the same banner in different states. Surely this adds to the cost of running a company and also contributes to the lack of real competition.

In my opinion, cost control, competition, elimination of fraud and real transparency would go a long way to addressing our health care issues and would cost very little to implement.

WHAT WE COULD BE DOING:

Cost control

As costs become prohibitive everyone is affected. Waste of resources in a hospital setting is the norm rather than the exception. With the current system there is no incentive for anyone to control costs.

Make it a patient-based system

That means prevention, protection, education, fairness, availability and affordability. Be able to buy insurance across state lines. Be able to buy coverage that suits your needs. Why cover someone for maternity when they have no way of getting pregnant? Allowing for basic diagnostic tests as part of your insurance premium makes sense. One mammogram a year for women, a PSA test every year for men, basic blood tests and a physical exam every year. The basics should be covered so that it encourages preliminary testing at no additional cost.

There should be transparency in pricing from insurance companies and hospitals and fair market competition

A possible start to this practice of transparency would be for hospitals to be required to post the costs of the 500 most common procedures that a hospital offers in its lobby, a "Sunshine List." The cost of a mammogram, ultrasound, blood test, chest X-ray, EKG, PSA test, etc. should not be under wraps but in the open. Only then do consumers get to make an informed choice. It is my belief hospitals don't want you to know the price of care, preferring instead to keep patients in the dark and making backroom deals with the insurance companies. It is time for everyone to come clean. Oddly even on the ubiquitous and powerful Internet it is hard to find the *cost* of procedures and treatment. And even when you make the effort and call an insurance company upfront they often don't tell you what your responsibility will be. They may tell you the percentage but again if you don't know the underlying cost the percentage is not decipherable. Believe me, they like it that way. It is time to get the price codes out in the open. A new Internet service, the Healthcare Blue Book, begins this process. But what is needed is a clear and accountable amount of what each provider specifically charges and not ballpark estimates.

Support 21st Century tools for education

We should have a math and science public television station that promotes learning about math and science 24/7. We should not forget the airwaves *belong* to the American people. Why can't there be classes on the airwaves all the time taught by the best professors and teachers in the world? The link between the broadcasters, the politicians and the money is doing systemic harm to our system of government. It is time we looked long and hard at the FCC and re-evaluated its role in not only entertainment but education and politics.

Real leadership on the fight against cancer in Washington

We are spending billions of dollars on scientific research but so many of those projects are pork-belly efforts having nothing to do with what Americans really care about. For example, they are building with millions of tax payer dollars a wine research facility on Long Island and doing so in the name of science. I like wine too but is that what we need to spend our money on when we are in a health crisis? Get rid of pork-belly spending. We can't afford it.

Support innovation

It is clear we are missing something when it comes to cancer. For all the lists of risk factors we don't know the triggers. If we really knew why then perhaps we could figure out how to prevent it. Surely the Cancer Genome Anatomy Project will be ground-breaking and full of answers, but it needs our support.

A national task force that evaluates our emergency room system

With many emergency rooms on "diversion" for long periods of time and unable to admit, we are clearly not in a position to handle a major crisis that may befall any major city. The current system with the uninsured being treated in an emergency room setting because it is their only alternative makes many emergency rooms across the country inadequate. These days everyone may have to wait for care. ER's often can't handle an emergency and *you* may very well be the emergency. If you want to evaluate the capacity of your hospital visit an emergency room and you will see the overflow. In 2008 I slept in a chair all night at Massachusetts General Hospital waiting for a room for my niece (who by the way had just been released that very day) because the hospital didn't have a bed for her (according to their computer). Meanwhile, I later found out the room she had just left was empty. There were gurneys with patients lining the halls and nearly every inch of the place was covered with bodies. And this is one of the finest hospitals in the country without a major disaster taking place. America, we have a serious emergency room problem.

Get every American covered with affordable insurance

Premiums need to be affordable. In my experience the only people that dismiss price as a factor are the ones that don't have to directly pay for it (getting coverage from an employer, a union or the government). In Bill 3590 the employer expense of health insurance will now be taxable to the employee (that will surely change the conversation). Allow and endorse open competition across state lines and allow for the insurance to travel with the person. A great example of the benefits of competition is what has happened in the phone industry over the last 20 years. There has been an explosion of choices, service and plans – the same can happen in health care.

Consider allowing doctors, especially specialists, to write any pro-bono work off their taxes

Currently hospitals insist that doctors and specialists (heart surgeons, oncology surgeons, plastic surgeons, orthopedic surgeons) who contract with the hospital must also treat their non-paying patients. Doctors are legally responsible for these patients whether or not they pay the bill. At the very least they should have a means of writing their skillful service off their federal income taxes.

Tort reform

Malpractice premiums have skyrocketed and the fear of lawsuits makes doctors practice defensive medicine – which isn't good for the patient or the doctor. This translates into unnecessary tests, higher costs and some doctors avoiding difficult cases. And on top of that most patients who need funds to live on because of mistakes or just bad outcomes aren't winning their lawsuits and are walking away with nothing. Lawyers are cherry picking the cases and only taking the ones where the payouts are huge. We have to get back to a common and decent way to handle human error. We must put fairness into the system and share the risk over the entire system. Otherwise, next time you (or your kids) go into an emergency room with a splinter in your eye there will be no eye surgeon available for you to see. They will have decided it isn't worth the liability. The advent of the "Apology movement" and a trend toward total transparency in acknowledging any medical errors is certainly a step in the right direction but we are a long way from honorable accountability and a compensation structure that is fair.

Health insurance redesign

And perhaps consider that health insurance should be redesigned and simplified for what it was originally intended to cover – the unexpected, catastrophic situations and not routine maintenance such as teeth cleaning As my friend David Goldhill wrote in an *Atlantic* piece in 2009, "Much of this enormous cost would simply disappear if we paid routine health care expenditures the way we pay for everything else – by ourselves." He points out that "for every two doctors in America we have one health insurance employee. In 2006 it costs $500 per person just to administer health insurance."

Reform, in my mind, does not mean we shouldn't pay doctors and nurses well. We should pay them exceptionally well for a number of reasons.

First, to help insure we get the best and the brightest to go into medicine and to reward them for their years of education and dedication. This is a field where the demand will only increase as the American population both increases and gets older. When many of the smartest and highest educated among us dismiss medicine as a career because the personal cost is too high and the compensation isn't commensurate with years of training relative to other endeavors perhaps we need to reevaluate our system. Selling credit default swaps has become much more profitable than becoming a doctor.

Second, the hours and working conditions in medicine will always be stressful and those who choose to enter this field need financial incentive. We need doctors to want to stay in an insurance system that works instead of opting out of the system and only be available to patients who pay cash.

During the negotiations of Bill 3590 some suggested that we should just expand the Medicare system. (The Medicare system takes care of anyone on Social Security or disability.) It is true at least there is a structure in place. And addressing the needs of folks that are in the 55-65 age bracket would certainly be helpful as the premiums this group pays are becoming increasing prohibitive. At least this primarily working demographic could pay into the system with their premiums. But Medicare is unsustainable in its present form, no less if we added people to the system. And reimbursements are not keeping up with actual costs. And obviously, we must eliminate the fraud. Medicare wasted 65 billion dollars in fraud in 2009. No wonder few have confidence in the government to run things efficiently.

Part of the new bill moves many onto the Medicaid rolls and has the states pick up the bill. But the states are having a hard time balancing their current budgets no less adding to their burden and they can't print money like the federal government has the ability to do. Again the full impact of the Affordable Care Act, from the dollars it will cost to the impact on America, has yet to see the light of day. But regardless I believe the medical community has to be more proactive about making the system transparent for consumers and not wait for the government to step in.

So while this is a political and philosophical argument that does not appear to be over, I wanted to offer *you,* the patient, some guidance on how to manage the current system if you have insurance.

WHAT YOU CAN DO:

Get personal

Get a name or two of someone at the insurance company with whom you can communicate. Explain your story to them. Ask this person to give you a number you can call if something comes up and you have a question. Write this name, number and address in your health notebook.

Organize

Create two health files or notebooks, one for your medical diagnosis, doctor notes, appointment dates, prescriptions, test results, notes on your symptoms and one for all of your insurance bills and doctor bills. They don't have to be perfect but if you organize it this way from the beginning you will have a better chance of recalling exactly what went on years later. Insurance bills come in months and sometimes years after the procedure and then doctor bills may arrive that are not covered by the insurance. It makes it easier to reconcile if you separate your health issues from your insurance issues when it comes to record keeping.

Communicate in writing

When dealing with the insurance companies and doctors over a bill correspond with them in writing. If you have an important conversation, follow up with a written note confirming the discussion. A fax is great for this because then you and they have a hard copy as a record. Again, it does not have to be formal but sending them a written copy of your complaint, problem or mistake on a bill goes a long way toward better communication and resolution. And make a copy for your records before you mail it to them. If you correspond by e-mail print your correspondence and save a copy in your file.

Negotiate

This is especially important if your doctor is not part of your health insurance plan. If you have special financial circumstances let the doctor know. If you need a payment plan they (the doctor or hospital) will be more likely to give you favorable terms if you tell them upfront what you can reasonably do. Also this gives you the cost information prior to the procedure.

Have it "authorized"

Make sure you have authorization from your insurance company before the procedure so it will pay for it. This isn't a guarantee that it will cover it but without it the insurer won't. The doctor may have to contact the insurance company for this but make sure you know that the authorization has been approved.

Get your doctor to be your advocate

If prescriptions are not automatically covered there is usually a phone number the doctor can call at the insurance company. This assurance by the doctor of the necessity of the drugs sometimes gets the insurance companies to cover what they may not ordinarily cover.

Consider out-of-state treatment

If you have more support or a better care-taking situation in another state your insurance company may cover you there and it may be better for you. For example, in Los Angeles many doctors I came across have opted out of the insurance system; however in Michigan, due to how most of them are paid, doctors are still in the Blue Cross system and I had a family support system there.

Read your policy and understand what you are entitled to

Know your deductible. You have to pay this *every* year. Know what your co pay is – you pay a certain percentage; the insurance company pays a certain percentage. And know at what dollar amount you are covered at 100% if at all per year. On many policies when you reach a certain amount for the year that you have paid out-of-pocket (not counting your insurance premiums) the insurer may have to cover you for 100% of the cost. This could impact the timing of optional or elective treatment. Since most of us don't reach this threshold normally it isn't something we are even aware of unless we review our insurance policies. Also know what the lifetime limit is (an issue that is also addressed in the new bill but may get adjusted). A million dollar lifetime limit sounds like a lot until you have a serious illness which can reach that threshold easily. See if you can increase your lifetime limit with minimum cost.

Investigate thoroughly doctors who are within your insurance system

Staying in-network helps keep the cost down. Going out-of-network can be expensive as cancer treatment often requires follow-up so you may be entering into a longer-term relationship than you first realized.

Get secondary coverage if you can afford it and it is available

If you have a spouse that can cover you with their plan, even if it means extra payments, in the long run it may be very beneficial. What one insurance doesn't pick up the other might on the same claim.

Ask for an itemized bill from the hospital

I was charged for an "operating room" when the procedure happened in a doctor's office. This kind of inaccuracy would show up on an itemized bill.

Keep a log of the services you received

If you are really concerned about the cost this is a good idea. If it sounds like too much work then the itemized bill should go a long way to making sure anything obviously incorrect is not on your bill.

Ask to be put on a payment plan

These can be adjusted to very low amounts, as little as $50 a month and much better than having them pressure you for the money with weekly phone calls. As I mentioned, one hospital billing office I dealt with actually said it was their policy "to call patients every week over an outstanding bill."

Get expert advice if necessary

If you find yourself overwhelmed by the insurance issues there are Claim Assistant Professionals (CAPs) who can be hired by the hour to sort it out. Try and get a good recommendation before hiring anyone.

Insurance issues don't go away. Deal with it yourself or ask for help from someone with the energy and expertise to organize it for you. And if you deal with it yourself, do it during the part of the day you have the most energy and patience. What insurance companies are hoping for is that you give up trying to get reimbursed when there is a dispute, especially if you have already paid for it with cash. In January 2006 I had a tattoo of a nipple done on my reconstructed breast. A year later I was still "communicating" with my insurance company about reimbursing me even though it had all the documentation. Fifteen months later they reimbursed me.

It seems wholly unfair that on top of being ill you should have to deal with uncooperative insurance companies but until something changes politically this system is all we have. To ignore the financial implications of this disease is to put yourself and maybe your family in jeopardy as even with insurance the expense can be overwhelming and you will need funds to deal with the future. Allocating your resources can be difficult but ignoring the implications of what cancer costs is not wise. If you don't ask for help in any other area this may very well be an area you need to ask for help.

If you have a problem with your insurance company and think it should cover a doctor or procedure that it is not covering due to out-of-network issues or excessive costs you do have the recourse to file a grievance with the insurer. If this is denied, you may be able to appeal the decision on the state level with the agency that oversees the insurance companies. In California this is the California Insurance Board, and other states have similar oversight agencies where you can send paperwork and make your case.

And also know cancer can create quite a dichotomy when it comes to your relationship with money. Money may feel both more important and less important in your life after you have been diagnosed. More important because you have a disease and need the financial ability to treat it (and pay your insurance premiums). But at the same time, money feels insignificant next to your health. Don't be surprised if your view of money changes with a breast cancer diagnosis.

14

Other Women

When you are diagnosed with breast cancer, you become an elder, no matter what your age.

– *Breast Cancer? Let me Check My Schedule*, Peggy McCarthy

When I hear breast cancer stories, nothing upsets me more than hearing the stories that involve a missed diagnosis or one mismanaged. Especially the ones where a woman feels that something isn't right, overcomes her fear, goes to get tested and is told everything is fine only to later find out her instincts were correct and the doctors were wrong. The time elapsed is critical as this is most often a silent and painless disease in its early stages. False assurances that nothing is wrong can lull one into a state of non-action and allow cancer to grow for years.

While I have shared my story of misdiagnosis, there are important lessons to be learned from the stories of other women too. Unique stories with common threads, and in this case the thread is not only breast cancer but misdiagnosis or mismanagement which turns out to be a costly mistake. And I mean costly in every way – emotionally, physically and financially.

CATHY NILON

Cathy Nilon lives in Seattle. In December 2004 she was 43. For seven years she had a lump that bothered her and was tender during her periods. She had mammograms and was told by four doctors it was a cyst.

In 2004 she had an ultrasound and then a stereotactic biopsy. It was invasive Stage 2b, estrogen receptor positive breast cancer. She has since had a double mastectomy, resection of the level two (deeper layer) lymph nodes on the one side and a hysterectomy. She had one lymph node involved and had chemo in January 2005. They inserted a port in her chest under the collarbone for the chemo, which due to her slim build hurt every time she hit it or rolled over at night although she admits it sure saved her veins from constant IV infusions and blood draws. At the time she had a four-year-old son and relatives living with her. Her mother, who stayed with her, was "a basket case" and was asked to leave. Her then boyfriend now husband, not sure what to do, bought a sports car. Eventually he turned out to be her "rock," missing work and staying up with her all night long. A vivid memory is the day she threw up in his precious car and almost lost her wig on I-5 going to treatment. To this day she hates that stinking car! Everyone coped as best they could. It was a tornado of emotions.

Her theory is that all her flying (she was in the shoe design business and went to Asia and Europe constantly, logging1.5 million miles in about 6 years) and the cosmic radiation she received contributed to her cancer. When you fly over 35,000 feet every four hours is equal to one chest X-ray. Without studies we will never know the full impact of cosmic radiation in aircraft. But, more importantly, she is another example of a woman feeling something is wrong and being told, for years, "It's nothing."

Cathy illustrated and wrote a children's book *Chemo Cat* about her experience with breast cancer. It was a way to help other families who are at a loss as to how to break the news of this illness to their children.

In early 2008, after her second reconstruction surgery using saline implants, she e-mailed me. "I have an infection in my breast. It is hot and pink, what do you think?" Turned out it was an infection that antibiotics cured but the terror in the e-mail that it could be IBC (Inflammatory Breast Cancer) or something else was apparent. The fear is always just below the surface.

Cathy is doing well in 2012.

JENNY APOLLONIO

Jenny Apollonio lives in Irvine, California with her three daughters and her husband. She is 52 as of this writing in 2012. She first found out she had cancer when she was 37 – but she too was misdiagnosed. Two years prior she found a lump and was told that it was "fibrocystic tissue" and therefore benign. She since has a more unique diagnosis: she has both ER positive cancer and is Her2 neu positive as well.

TIP: While it is rare to have more than one distinct pathology, it can occur.

Her perspective is, "Doctors are not God. If you aren't satisfied with their answers look elsewhere." Her original anger is still not far from the surface. It was first suggested that she have a stem cell transplant. A second opinion told her to have neo-adjuvant chemo and then surgery which is what she opted for. Since then it has been determined that the current stem cell transplant protocol is not effective for breast cancer.

Jenny has gone through three rounds of chemo – in 1998, 2000, and 2002. "It is awful. If anyone tells you differently they are lying but you do get through it." She never had a port installed. She had a mastectomy and tram flap reconstruction.

When I asked her what was the lowest point she told me, "It was after the first diagnosis, chemo, surgery, more surgery and being cancer-free for two years and then being told it had come back...my first recurrence." In her mind she had decided that she was cancer-free – that if it came back it was a death sentence. That she had given it her best shot. Here is the hopeful part...that was twelve years ago.

Jenny has three daughters. When she was first diagnosed they were 7, 5 and 1. What she said to the girls was simple but what they could understand. She told them, "I have something in my breast that isn't suppose to be there and they were going to give me really strong medicine that will make me feel not so good and my hair will fall out. But you know what? When it grows back again, that means I'm getting better."

Her husband offered support and strength and "went to every weird healing thing I dragged him to. He was great. He always let me know I was going to be okay and it was never an option or discussed that I wasn't."

Two of her coping mechanisms came in the form of meditation and visualization tapes. One tape in particular was by Carl Simonton. For her they were a great help when it came to sleeping and feeling some power over the disease. And she accepted help from friends.

Jenny said, "I kind of lived in denial most of the time and never made a big deal when I was treated. I had little ones to deal with so I carried on as usual as much as possible. I still helped in school, threw birthday parties and car-pooled. Then secretly barfed my brains out."

When I asked her what she did to stay vigilant she said, "I have a lot of help. I am currently on Herceptin. It's an infusion every three weeks and this has been going on for over three years. I have blood work done every time and Pet/CT scans every year. I guess you would say my doctor is vigilant. You are never the same as before cancer. It is always there."

As of 2012 Jenny is doing well and still being treated.

TIP: Herceptin was developed as a way to "turn off" the HER2/Neu gene. It is an antibody to the HER2/Neu protein. If you are HER2/Neu positive this may be a treatment for you. It has certainly been a miracle drug for women who are HER2/Neu positive.

PEDEN FITZHUGH

When I first met Peden it was at our monthly breast cancer lunch – she was bald, going through chemo and had a blue head scarf on. Her smile was huge. My first few thoughts were, "How can someone be so sick, so beautiful, so young and have breast cancer?" Breast cancer doesn't care.

Peden was 31 when she discovered her breast cancer. As she says, "I woke up in the middle of the night and then, since I was awake, decided to give myself a breast self exam. I had done it a few times in my life but certainly not regularly. Then I thought I felt something, so I promptly freaked out and could not go back to sleep. In the morning I Googled some information that told me young women's breasts can feel particularly lumpy during different parts of their cycle. I went to see my primary physician; she didn't feel anything but suggested I have an ultrasound." And then, what happened to Peden I think happens to a lot of women. She did not have confidence in her original thought that "she felt something" and never made the ultrasound appointment. For five months the lump grew until one day it was noticeable from the outside of her breast. As she puts it, "After seeing dimpling in my breasts under a fluorescent light I decided to schedule the ultrasound appointment." After the ultrasound a mammogram was recommended and then a biopsy of the site. It was confirmed that it was cancer. She was ER and PR positive and Her-2nue positive.

She then had another all too common experience. She got two sets of treatment recommendations. One California team of doctors advised double mastectomy, followed by six rounds of chemo, a year of Herceptin and five years of tamoxifen. Her Georgia team of doctors was more interested in conserving her breast tissue and recommended chemo pre-surgery in order to shrink the tumor (which was 3-5cm long), followed by either a lumpectomy or a mastectomy and then Herceptin and tamoxifen. She decided to opt for the more aggressive surgery options and had the double mastectomy with reconstruction.

When I asked her about the chemo she said, "I really hated it. I felt a lot of fatigue and nausea although continued to work throughout. Food tasted like cardboard and salting made it taste metallic." She was very glad she had the port in her arm for the infusions.

Her lowest point came one day after her first chemo, feeling listless and not knowing which medication would help. As she was taking a bath she realized that she was going to have to submit to feeling this bad five more times. It was a terrible feeling, not knowing when it would end and knowing it was going to happen again. She understood then, for the first and only time in her life, why someone would want to take her own life. The acuteness of the depression when you get this news and have to take drastic measures to deal with it – mastectomy and chemo – can take you down.

What proved to be a real blessing is that she started dating a guy two weeks before she was diagnosed and to quote her, "He has been pretty awesome. We took it slow in the beginning as we were still getting to know each other and I tried not to rely on him too much during that time. But having a guy by your side who loves you and tells you you're sexy even when you are bald, pale and putting on 15 pounds is of tremendous emotional support." *Can we clone him?*

When I asked what she wanted women to know about breast cancer she said, "I want women to know that it's absolutely possible to get breast cancer even if you've eaten your antioxidants and worn aluminum-free deodorant – if you've done everything 'right' you may still be at risk." And being under 40 is no insurance that you will not get this disease.

On the subject of telling people, Peden chose to be the one to share the news with a wide range of people. For her being open about it helped her on a lot of levels. First she had lots of companions who would go with her to the doctors and would sit with her during treatment. She had a large number of people praying for her. And she found talking to people about it therapeutic. She had a therapist but, as she explains, "I never had to wait a week to bring something up with her – I felt free to discuss my feelings as I was feeling them with whomever might be around. This freedom really helped me from feeling stressed and overwhelmed."

And she wanted people to know that just because the most grueling part of the medical treatment may be over, there are still side effects to deal with. Physical fatigue, emotional stress and processing what just happened takes a lot of bandwidth. It may not be obvious but she is still very much "in process" when it comes to her breast cancer. She knows full-well life will never be the same.

She is mad that at 31 she got cancer and, in her words, "It hurts a lot to think that the choice to have children may have been taken away from me." And she is also worried about a recurrence, of course. The only worry she doesn't have is that she found out short hair suits her. I told you, young and beautiful.

As of 2012 Peden is doing well. And, great news, she is engaged to be married.

PAM CERRUTI

Pam Cerruti is 56 as of this writing in 2012 and a family law attorney living in Montclair, New Jersey. She and I have been great friends for over 40 years. She has the energy of a 25-year-old and running 3 miles a day is a regular event for her.

She found her "lump," or as she describes it, something that "felt like the head of a pin" in the shower while doing a breast self exam in 1997. She immediately went to the breast doctor who did a clinical breast exam, a mammogram and an ultrasound. She was told nothing worrisome was found and to come back in six months. Four weeks later the breast doctor reconsidered and said Pam had been on her mind and she wanted to see her again. This time when the doctor felt the lump it had clearly grown in 4 weeks. Pam had a lumpectomy that week and was told it was benign.

Three days later she was getting "frantic" calls from her doctor saying she had not read the last page of the pathology report and that Pam had Stage 4 Invasive Ductal Carcinoma. The doctor informed her she needed to do more surgery.

Pam started researching it herself and found Dr. Michael Lagious in California, who specializes in the forensics of the breast. She made arrangements for the slides of her original biopsy to be sent to him. He concluded that the second diagnosis was incorrect, that she had DCIS, Ductal carcinoma in-situ, not invasive carcinoma and that she should have another lumpectomy to assure clear margins and have radiation. Pam did all that and all is well 15 years later.

The lessons she takes away? Surround yourself with people who love you and make you laugh, don't just take what any doctor tells you and run with it but instead get a second opinion and keep physically fit (she walks the talk) because your body has enough to do to keep the cancer away.

Pam continues to run and keep active and has added NCAA basketball referee to her C.V. As of 2012 she is doing very well.

MARY ROSENBERG

Mary Rosenberg is on the front lines of what breast cancer treatment can bring. As a lymphedema specialist and physical therapist, she sees the battle-weary every day. Her clients may have fought the cancer but now they are dealing with swelling and discomfort the treatment and surgery may have left behind. As a breast cancer survivor, Mary knows all the emotions that go along with a breast cancer diagnosis.

She too was told by her doctor when she first found the lump "not to worry," that it is probably just fibroadenoma. The biopsy proved otherwise.

During dinner with her family she got a phone call from her doctor, "You have cancer." That night she had to take her son to his bar mitzvah lesson at the temple (life doesn't stop). When she saw the rabbi's secretary she "lost it." The shock and fear of the unknown made her break down.

She later found out she was Stage 1, ER and PR positive but at the time didn't know if she was going to live or die. She was initially told by the first medical oncologist to have a bilateral mastectomy and chemotherapy. This was from a doctor whose wife had had the same treatment two years before. She changed doctors and instead had three lumpectomies followed by a mastectomy. She was one of the first patients in a study of sentinel node biopsies.

Mary was lucky to have a very supportive husband, family and friends. They made her feel like it was her birthday, every day. It was clear as I talked to her that her husband in particular was her rock – unconditional in his support, researching the disease online for her and telling her it didn't matter to him if she had reconstruction or not – her choice – he was going to be just as turned on by her with or without a right breast.

She wishes insurance companies would just pay the claims without contesting obvious charges and that Medicare would approve bandages and compression garments for lymphedema because without the garments management of this condition is ineffective.

For her, sharing the news she had breast cancer helped alleviate the burden of the disease. She would like women to know that early detection is so important. Her work has proven to be healing not only to her clients but for herself. Being able to reach out and contribute to the community has given her life more purpose.

As of 2012 Mary is doing well.

WHERE ELSE MY LIFE HAS BEEN TOUCHED BY BREAST CANCER.

HELEN CAKE

My Aunt Sis was a favorite great aunt. She was gay when it wasn't acceptable to be so. A secretary most of her life, she could type 120 words a minute on an Underwood. She had a complete (radical) mastectomy in the 1960s. In those days they took all your muscles and lymph nodes: everything. When I was 17-years-old I asked her about her cancer. She showed me her scar in her bedroom in Manhattan Beach, California in 1972. My knees buckled and I almost passed out. It was the most horrific mutilation I had ever seen. The single right breast gone, the area now concave and the ugly jagged red scar went from her collarbone to her belly button. I had no idea that was the result of what it meant to have breast cancer in 1960.

Because surgeons had taken all the lymph nodes on that side of her body near the cancer she wore an arm brace/compression garment to keep the swelling down from the severe lymphedema. She would certainly have been amazed at the advances made since then, had she been able to see me after my surgery. She never had reconstruction and would occasionally curse the prosthetic (too darn hot) she wore for appearances sake.

An admitted alcoholic, and the first person I knew helped by AA, she became aware of her problem with alcohol when her routine after work had to include a stop at the liquor store, not daring to go home unless she was certain alcohol was waiting for her. She always thought, and told me often, there was a connection between her drinking and getting breast cancer. This was a connection no one was making at the time but now high alcohol consumption is considered a definite risk factor. She died in 1980 after a long battle.

"GERRY"

"Gerry" (not her real name) was my mother's friend and a member of her "Club." My mother, Pat Armenti, had an unusual and remarkable group of friends. These women had been friends since high school and met every Tuesday night (and still do). They had, what growing up in my house was fondly known as, Club.

It was a ritual no one messed with...not husbands, not kids. There were 11 of them in the beginning. If five "girls" were available then Club was on. The "girls" would rotate houses, hosting with pineapple upside down cake and homemade brownies. They would arrive at around 7:00 P.M. with Club actually starting at 7:30 P.M. Soft drinks and snacks would be served. Then they would sit down and play cards for pennies. They wouldn't get to a quarter in the pot until the end of the night right before cake and coffee were served.

I loved it when Club was at our house and the "girls" made me feel like I was part of it. I remember being so small that when I stood at the dining room table I had to stand on my tip toes to see the faces of the cards. And on the last hand they would deal me in.

When Gerry was diagnosed with breast cancer it rocked the Club but they held together. The fear and the compassion went through the whole group. Gerry was the Club girl that maybe wouldn't be there on Tuesday night. She was getting treatments or too tired. "What happened at the doctor?"The women would always talk about her, hushed and sad, remembering her in the conversation like prayer. Gerry bravely fought breast cancer for over 20 years.

TIP: This may surprise you but ask what would be the treatment if you had a more severe case. It *does not* mean you should have that treatment but asking for the information gives you the chance to make a more informed decision with your doctor. This is hard because the tendency is to want to be optimistic about your prognosis and not explore a more advanced case. Generally you do not want to know a worst case scenario but you deserve to know what your options are, even if you ultimately choose with your doctor a more conservative path. For example, a sentinel node biopsy is not usually offered to women with DCIS even if they have a lumpectomy or a mastectomy whereas if you had

invasive cancer it would be standard protocol to see if it had spread. And once the mastectomy is performed mapping the lymph nodes is no longer an option. Information is power and can provide treatment options you never knew existed.

Lessons

I think the lesson I have learned is there is no substitute for paying attention.

– Diane Sawyer

So there are some basic lessons I have taken away from this experience. They have come at a high cost and I would like to share them with you.

1) ***Get the test if needed.*** Your fear may be hard to manage but avoiding a test because of it is not smart. There is a correlation between early detection and survival rates. If it is found only in the breast there is the chance (not a guarantee) that it hasn't traveled and it can be removed. Once it has been found in the lymph system and beyond (bones, liver, lung, brain) the entire nature of the disease changes. It becomes "systemic," which means it has infiltrated the system of the body and requires a much more intense protocol.

2) ***Read the reports and ask questions about the diagnosis.*** No one is more interested in your health than you. Don't expect the doctors and nurses to make you the priority. You may not be able to interpret everything on a pathology report but you can gain an understanding of a lot of it and sometimes obvious things get missed by doctors. You deserve an explanation and reading it together with your doctor will diminish the chances of something important being overlooked. And send a copy or have them send a copy to your general practitioner – the more people who read the report the less likely something obvious will get missed.

3) Don't listen to good news if your body is telling you something different. You know your body better than anyone. If you think something is wrong check it out until you have exhausted all the tests available. And if you feel "good" don't ignore a bad diagnosis and assume the test must be wrong because you feel fine. Cancer is stealthy and deadly and most often painless in its early stages. Waiting or procrastinating is foolish if the empirical facts tell you otherwise.

4) ***Talk and share if you want.*** It is your body and your health and you get to choose whom you share the information with and how much. There are no rights and wrongs around this – it is your choice to make.

5) ***You have to be your own advocate with your doctors, with the hospital and with the entire nursing staff or have someone that can do it for you.*** If something doesn't feel right speak up. Know who you are and what you can tolerate. And if you can't advocate for yourself having someone advocate for you is sometimes the best gift anyone can give you. Don't be in a hospital alone as pain medicine and procedures can make you incoherent and unable to express yourself. This is not a luxury but a necessity.

6) ***Ask ahead of time what this will cost.*** Sometimes you can negotiate a reduced fee in advance – that goes for doctors and hospitals. Ultimately you will be responsible for the final accounting after insurance companies pay their portion. And check around for what it may cost at another facility.

7) *Treat yourself to as much self-care as you can give yourself.* You may be determined to do more...be okay with doing less. Have a massage, get your nails done, take a soothing bath, ask for help with the kids, meditate, get your hair done, take a walk in nature, play with your pet, have sex if you feel like it, take a nap, exercise, read a book and give to others in a way that benefits you rather than drains you. Doing something every day that feeds you and clears your head is worthwhile. Diversions are welcomed. You don't need permission...just do it.

8) *Stay vigilant.* Yes, it is hard to keep getting tested. There is nothing fun about going to the oncologist, having ultrasounds and MRIs but it is the only way to know what is going on at a cellular level. You have to make it a priority – this means your time, your resources, and your energy. Life just changed and this is no time to put your head in the sand.

9) *Have fun, laugh and do what you love with whom you love.* So you just got a shocking wake-up call that this life isn't going to last forever. Some days you will feel good and my suggestion is to "just say yes." Do what makes life joyful and eliminate as much of the extra stuff and people you can. Have the people in your life that really love and support you and be okay with letting go of the ones that can't be there for you. I always wanted to go to the Kentucky Derby. In 2007 I went with my good friend Lynn. It was, as my great-grandmother, Mimi, would say "grand." Get clear about what you don't want to miss and do it now.

10) *Take your sleep seriously.* Sleep is very restorative and I believe a time of deep healing. While seemingly at rest your body continues to perform the necessary functions of breathing, digestion, brain function, swallowing, etc. – which are all essential to your staying alive. Your body is also resetting, recharging and healing that which needs healing or at least it is trying to. Get a comfortable bed and protect your sleep.

11) *Meditate on gratitude.* Hard to do when life is unfair. However, negativity is throwing good energy after bad and you only have so much energy. Be grateful for whatever good you have and have had in your life and grateful for what the not-so-good can teach you and accept it all. In the popular book *Eat, Pray, Love* the guru's suggestion is to "smile when meditating." Being present *in gratitude* can offer you a perspective that is focused on the spirit, where there is no cancer, rather than the body.

Conclusion

Your life will not be defined by what you get but by what you give away.

The only good news I can think of about a cancer diagnosis is it gives you permission to write a memoir at any age. Even so, as I was writing this book, I often wondered if I should continue. Is my perspective relevant for others? Is it informative? Are there too many breast cancer books on the market already? And podcasts and blogs? Maybe everyone already knows all this. Self-doubt, the bane of every writer.

But then another story would be on the nightly news, or I would read a message board where a woman newly diagnosed would be asking for help, or I would get an e-mail from a well-meaning girlfriend with somewhat misleading information (such as legislation regarding mastectomies and a designated amount of time you should be in the hospital – something I feel should *not* be legislated but left up to patients and their doctors to determine (and the NBCC agrees) or I would talk to someone being treated and wonder why she didn't know about sentinel node biopsy or I would hear once again about all the "advances they are making" and think "that just isn't good enough and it isn't the whole story." And I would again sit at my computer and write. I would also think about all the women I know that have breast cancer and especially the women who have allowed me to share part of their stories with you. Their blood, sweat and tears (literally) needed to be documented.

Like I said, for me it will always come down to a single woman. The woman who this very day has to face the news that life, as she knew it, has changed. I picture her frozen in a hospital parking lot after talking to her doctor. I know she didn't hear anything after the words, "You have breast cancer." I see her glazed face and her need for answers, support, information and hope. Whom does she call? Did she stop by the book store on the way home from the doctor or will she search the computer in the middle of the night desperate to get informed? That while she has heard so much about breast cancer, maybe even had it in her family or experienced it with a friend, until they say it to you it can be just another word. When they say *you* have it, it is like a noun becoming a verb. *Cancer*. It is on the move and it requires action. So if even a single woman faced with the diagnosis found this book comforting, informative or inspiring then it was worth it. It was worth the time, the painful reflection, the exposure and the lack of privacy.

The landscape is not just replete with women who have gone through cancer but with decimated families as well. Cancer is a family illness. It takes too much to be considered otherwise. And for me, it is also about the children. When they lose a parent it damages their present life and, without at least a cure, their future is at risk.

As I was writing this book, Elizabeth Edwards lost her brave battle with breast cancer. On December 7, 2010, she died at the age of 61 with young children yet to raise. As a breast cancer survivor when you hear of a breast cancer death it isn't just a tragic news story but a reminder of how notoriously relentless this disease can be. Even though you may have no personal knowledge of the person who died you have a visceral connection to the struggle. It gets your attention and holds it and you replay it in your head. You can't help but ask, "What was that like for her?" This is the time when you need to find joy in something. Something that will raise you up rather than pull you into a state of mind that makes the outcome appear inevitable.

All this makes me examine the realities. It shouldn't be hard or expensive to get a mammogram. It shouldn't be a fight to have an MRI if that is what is needed. It shouldn't be insignificant to lessen someone's pain before a biopsy. It shouldn't be outrageously expensive to have reconstructive surgery. You shouldn't have to do battle with your insurance company while you are fighting cancer. To deny people palliative care because they can't pay for it when pain relief is within our ability is cruel. And to ignore end of life issues and not bring compassion to those dying, especially the ones who find themselves alone, is not being our best. To be harassed by hospital bill collectors while you can barely lift your head from the pillow seems un-American.

I believe for the most part that if you know better and *have the capacity*, you do better. So I would ask you if this book ends up in your hands and you are in a position to do something about any of this, please do it. Small steps add up. Change the hospital policy if you work for a hospital, review the insurance company's way of dealing with cancer patients if you work for an insurer, promote legislation that is right for patients if you are a citizen or legislator but, of course, talk to patients and doctors first if you are a legislator as we do not need just more laws but smarter ones. And if you are a doctor or a health care professional understand that it isn't just a procedure you are performing on a patient. It is more than that, much more.

If you are a health care professional know *what you do* is just as important as *how you do it.* You are dealing with someone whose life has been threatened by an unscrupulous and notorious enemy. One that is sneaky, consuming, relentless and stealth. You may be the technician conducting what looks to you like a routine mammogram or ultrasound but I assure you, if the patient has been diagnosed with cancer in the past, nothing is routine. Because on that day, when the patient first found out she had cancer, that day also looked like every other day, until it wasn't.

In 2007 Miles Levin, a young man with cancer who became well-known due to his brave and thoughtful response to it, asked his high school graduating class to consider what is one's responsibility if you draw the "long end of the stick." I don't know how long the stick is that I have drawn. Will I die from breast cancer and if so when? Questions that can't be answered from this vantage point. What I do know is that we all have a responsibility to use our experience to, at the very least, speak up and articulate what we have learned and what we really believe in.

Kerry Kennedy wrote a book, *Speak Truth to Power.* It is about voices speaking out to the powers of control. This is my attempt to "*speak truth to power.*"The power of the insurance companies to raise premiums and limit what they cover and then cover things you don't need and charge you for it, the power of hospitals that don't tell you what something costs, the power of the accepted standard of care and the status quo that falls short, the manipulation of the data to sell drugs, the arrogance and insensitivity of some nurses and doctors, the power of our elected officials and the lobbies that court them.

As a patient I can't get a pain pill without a doctor's prescription. I am an adult. I own my own business. I can fly across the country or around the world without asking permission. I can buy a quart of vodka, ride a motorcycle and spend all my money buying lottery tickets but as a cancer patient I can't give myself a single pain pill without a doctor saying it is okay. They have a lock on it. That comes with accountability. And my point of view is that we should give others only minimal control over our lives and monitor it very, very carefully.

Many of the breast cancer books I have read paint a medically PC picture. Maybe because they were written by doctors looking for research grants with positions they need to protect or maybe they were written by women who survived and were so grateful to their doctors that they don't want to criticize. In any case, they don't seem to question the insurance companies, the protocols, the psychological treatment, the hospital procedures and the lack of progress.

Yes, there has been progress but as a society we have spent billions and have been fighting cancer for decades. I personally think the tools in the tool shed are not as cutting edge as one would expect after all the dollars and the time. So I have a more defiant voice and it is 100% intentional. As Dr. Christine Winthrop would say, this is the time to, "Do it on purpose and play it out loud." I always come back to the same thought. When are they going to figure out what causes this disease and prevent it, and in the meantime find humane and compassionate protocols to manage it?

Fear is paralyzing. Just today, a woman I have known for 20 years and ran into at a work function asked me what else I have been doing. I told her I was writing a book about breast cancer. She said, "I'm going for a mammogram tomorrow. My doctor found a lump. Gosh, don't know why I told you. I haven't told anyone. I haven't even told my husband yet." I gave her my home phone number and told her, "You may have some questions, call me if you want." It again made it clear how the fear stops women in their tracks. I know there are others reading this who haven't told anyone yet. It's okay, you need time to adjust to even the possibility; it is that scary.

Cancer so easily consumes everything; you have to hold on to life, because the cancer (the diagnosing of it, treating it and living with the fear of it) is constantly fighting for the all oxygen in the room. I found it is better not to make it a constant focus and the only thing that has my attention. Writing this book has made that harder but it was a consequence of speaking up.

Being woken up in the middle of the night from breast cancer may be unique to me. I've never heard of that happening to another women so please don't expect it to happen to you. However, I have heard women say, "I knew something was wrong and I ignored it." Or, "I knew something was wrong but they kept on saying it was nothing." That is the message here. If your body is trying to tell you something, don't ignore it...while sleeping or awake. I have even heard of a woman after a double mastectomy who still felt the tumor and while doctors didn't believe her at first she proved to be right. They had missed it.

I needed to write about my experience because I needed to claim it – the unreal part of it, the pain, the frustration and the fortunate part that I was able to listen to that sometime distant but powerful inner voice that wouldn't let a wrong, clear diagnosis satisfy me. My intention was to separate each moment so that I could move through it and not have it continue to run me. Like a tissue sample, I had to slice it up and look at it under the microscope. Did I do the right thing, what is the lesson and more importantly who else could be helped by this?

While I had a serious disease I was also very lucky that it wasn't worse, that I didn't take things at face value and suppress my intuition. And while that part of the road is behind me I still remember the way and I needed to post a sign at the entrance. "Warning – all is not what it appears."

If you have ever been driving on a country road alone in a winter storm, lost, at night, not certain if you will get home and hoping the gas and the car hold up...that is kind of what a breast cancer diagnosis is like. You are leaning forward, trying to get a better look at the road, tension in your shoulders, heart-rate elevated, aware of the dark and the danger. Now when I get lost I try to remember how different the same road looks in the sunshine. I wish for you lots of days in sunshine.

So here I am 16 years later. I think I am a bit wiser and I know I am feistier. Not that I wasn't feisty before (ask anyone who knows me) but don't mess with me now! Don't give me a needle that is too big or tell me that I can't see the monitor when you ultrasound me, or tell me I don't need a biopsy when I think I do or give me a dirty look when I say don't go any tighter on the mammogram machine or overcharge me. I'm a cancer veteran and I won't have it.

That said, I am also very grateful for the skill and compassion I did receive from medical staff along the way. Some of you make Superman and Superwoman appear mortal.

About the Author

Susan Armenti has enjoyed a remarkable career – several of them. At 26, she flew up the ranks of prestigious Condé Nast to become the production manager of *Vogue* magazine in New York City working for both Grace Mirabella and Anna Wintour. Following years in magazine publishing she moved west to Hollywood and worked for Columbia Studios and Warner Bros. and then as a film agent with the William Morris Agency in Beverly Hills, where she represented actors such as Elizabeth Taylor and packaged and sold movies. She has written several screenplays. *Sensation in the Night, Waking up to Breast Cancer* is her first non-fiction book. She owns Holmby Park Realty, is an avid equestrian and a 16 year cancer veteran.

Pink Ribbon

Where did it come from? We all know of the Pink Ribbon symbol of breast cancer. It came into being as a result of the partnership between Evelyn H. Lauder (1936-2011) from Lauder Cosmetics and Alexandra Penny from *Self* magazine, a Condè Nast Publication. It first became the symbol of breast cancer in October 1992 when it appeared on the cover of *Self*. Evelyn H. Lauder founded the Breast Cancer Research Foundation which has raised over 200 million dollars for breast cancer research.

From 1979 to 1984 I worked at *Vogue*, eventually becoming the production manager. I originally got the job because my boss, Linda Rice, was moving to a more corporate position as Condè Nast expanded its list of magazines. *Self* magazine was the first one in the expansion. Ironic for me that the infamous Pink Ribbon would first show itself on a magazine that had already had such a huge impact on my life.

Acknowledgments

Without many of these people in my life this book would not have happened. And when you add breast cancer you have a lot of people to thank. They all have my lasting gratitude.

My parents, Fred and Pat Armenti, who knew none of this in their lifetime but everything now. Nothing takes the place of great parents. And my guardian angels including all those in the Armenti family as well as Helen Cake, Helen "Mimi" Smith, Connie and John Comfort and Lee Cake.

My entire family, especially my always amazing brother, Dr. Frederick Armenti, without whom there may have never been a 2012 for me no less a book. And especially my nieces, Amanda Armenti and Monica Armenti, and my brother Tom, Noreen, Kent and Brooke Armenti. Also special thanks to Sue Cake, June, Sean and Charlie Comfort, Norma and Joe Comfort, Jennifer, Jodi and Michael Comfort, Hope Armenti, Carmen V. Armenti, Melinda Armenti, Nick and Marie Armenti, Marea and Ted Dumbauld, Erma and Bobby Candelori, Chris and Carmen Armenti, Charles and JoAnne Armenti, Debbie and Anthony Armenti, Phyllis and Carmen Armenti and Joseph Armenti.

And to my friends and others who made a greater contribution than I can measure. Michael Lambert, who was able to be there for some of the scary parts. Pam Cerruti, for 40 years of friendship and for sharing her story. Nancy Fromm who knows what consistent love really does to the spirit. It heals it. Also Tricia Catanese Adler,

Christopher White and Donna Grovesnor, Ellen Bloom, Paul "Hamilton" Magid, Patti and Peter Matthews, Gary Niels, Nancy Dunn, Jeff Michael and Evan, Shari Geffen, Dr. Kathleen Mojas, Kim Hahn, Robert Masello, Sarah Vienot, Luci Saha, Irene Hill, Linda Lee Marent, Lynn Ziegenfuss, Will Hemminger, Morgan Mason, Christine Danzo, Isabelle Gibert, Richard and Dorsey Renaldo, Richard and Daphna Ziman, Maria Conchita Alonso, Danielle Guttman Klein, Mary Lambert, Alexi Dureck and Colin Fulford, Anna Diaz, Deborah Raffin, Susan Ringler, Anna Marie Kostura, Lorne Pollock, Karen Glasser, Hailey Sweet, Joan Harrison, Julie and Rich Powers, Dave Bair, Allan and Elaine Rich, Dr. R. Trigg McClellan, Bonnie Adams, Dana DeVorzon, Beverly Retseck, Jacqui Lofaro and Deborah Kooperstein, Fadia and Mick De Falco. And Eddie and Denise Bernstein, a match made in heaven – thanks for letting me take the credit.

Others who made a difference – Maryanne Reisng who took me drains and all out to lunch when company was more important than food. All the "Club girls" who taught me in my childhood more about female friendship by example than any book ever written. And to all the brave women in the BC lunch group and to Bonnie Schut who keeps it all going.

And to those who supported me and the book my sincere thanks. Heidi Kummer, M.D., and Karl Breuing, M.D. Heidi, my angel, who helped guide me and this book and Karl for offering your expertise on breast reconstruction. Elsie Levin, M.D., who allowed me to take photos of her Boston Breast Diagnostic Center. George Retseck, for your wonderful illustrations. Laurie Drake, for your loving phone call early on which made me know it was important and resonated and for your eagle eye. Gretchen Morgenson, for our friendship and your unwavering support. Michael Gendelman, Katherine Woodward Thomas and Arnold Goodman for your encouraging words.

Gloria Emerson was a friend and winner of the National Book Award and the only female *New York Times* correspondent during the Vietnam War. When I visited her in her home on Mercer Street in Princeton, New Jersey, many years ago and looked into her study where she wrote, I said, "Is that where you work?" She responded instantly, "No, that is the torture room." I thought of her often as I wrote and it made me realize that writing is hard but no reason to give up.

And for inspiration, Mike Smith and Zenyatta – champions always and forever. Zenyatta confirmed that which is extraordinary can always, even after breast cancer, enter my life.

And the doctors who I know did and continue to do their best – Dr. Steiner, Dr. Saha, Dr. Hayden, Dr. Rudnick, Dr. Van Scoy-Mosher, Dr. Alghanem and Dr. Dinome, thank you for your care.

And for the women who know this walk and let me share their stories and their steps so that others would be informed – Jenny, Cathy, Linda, Peden and Mary.

Resources

Lance Armstrong Foundation
www.Livestrong – Great site for general cancer information.

American Cancer Society
www.AmericanCancerSociety – 1-800-ACS-2345. Check out its Reach for Recovery Program. You will get to meet and talk with others who have gone through breast cancer. They will give you bras that work well after surgery.

National Cancer Institute 1-800-4-CANCER
www.cancer.gov.

Triple Negative Breast Cancer Foundation
www.tnbcfoundation.org
Website dedicated to Triple negative breast cancer.

Young Survivor Coalition
www.youngsurvival.org
Group that focuses on young (under 40) breast cancer patients and survivors

Fertile Hope
www.fertilehope.com
Fertility and cancer.

www.cancer.org

www.lymphnet.org
National Lymphedema Network

National Coalition for Cancer Survivorship
www.canceradvocay.org

Susan G. Komen Breast Cancer Foundation
www.Komen.org
1-800-IM-AWARE

National Breast Cancer Coalition
www.breastcancerdeadline2020.org
An advocacy group interested in promoting dialogues that focus on facts and funding. Offers training for breast cancer advocacy.

National Alliance of Breast Cancer Organization
www.nabcc.com

Wellness Community
www.thewellnesscommunity.org

KidsCope
www.kid-support.org

Breast Cancer Org.
www.breastcancer.org.
Web based non-profit for information.

Books and Magazines

Dr. Susan Love Breast Book by Susan M. Love, M.D. with Karen Linsey

Breast Cancer, Real Answers, Real Questions by Dr. David Chan, M.D.

M.D. Anderson Cancer Care Series, Breast Cancer by Kelly K. Hunt, Geoffrey L. Robb, Eric A. Strom, Naoto T. Ueno

What Your Doctor May Not Tell You About Breast Cancer by John R. Lee, MD, David Zava, PhD, and Virginia Hopkins

Uplift Secrets of the Sisterhood of Breast Cancer Survivors by Barbara Delinsky

Mamma Said There Would Be Days Like This: A Twelve Step Guide to Surviving Mastectomy by Karen Klein

The Victoria Secret Catalog Never Stops Coming by Jeannie Nash

Living in the Post Mastectomy Body: Learning to Live in and Love Your Body Again by Rebecca L. Zuckweiler

After Mastectomy: Healing Physically and Emotionally by Rosiland Benedet

Why I Wore Lipstick to My Mastectomy by Geralyn Lucas

Pretty is What Changes by Jessica Queller

Taking Care of Your "Girls": A Breast Health Guide for Girls, Teens and In-Betweens by Dr. Marisa Weiss and Isabel Friedman

B.O.O.B.S.: A Bunch of Outrageous Breast Cancer Survivors Tell Their Stories of Courage, Hope and Healing by Ann Fisher

I'm Too Young To Have Cancer by Beth Leibson-Hawkins

Positively Pink by Jennifer A. Tom

Choices in Breast Cancer Treatment, edited by Kenneth D. Miller, MD, Johns Hopkins Press Health Book

Places Of the Soul by Christopher Day

Breast Cancer Husband: How to help Your Wife (And Yourself) through Diagnosis, Treatment and Beyond by Marc Silver

The Breast Reconstruction Guidebook by Kathy Steligo

Second Opinion by Dr. Jerome Groopman

It's Not about the Bike by Lance Armstrong

Heal A magazine about healing.

Dreaming in Hindi: Coming Awake in Another Language by Katherine Russell Rich

The Red Devil: To Hell with Cancer...and Back by Katherine Russell Rich

Shopping

www.mastectomy.com Mastectomy.com 1-888-966-7068. A variety of bras and breast forms. Swimwear and sleepwear.

www.Jodee 3100 North 29th Ave., Hollywood, Fla. 99020 (800) 423-9038

www.TomsofMaine.com Tom's of Maine, P.O Box 710, Kennebunk, ME 04043

www.healingthreads.com Kimono-type hospital gowns. 1-877-647-3900

www.stillyoufashions.com 336-282-9816. Stylish sleepwear and bras.

www.astrazeneca.com Emla (numbing cream) Astra Pharmaceuticals.

www.gebauerco.com Pain Ease (numbing spray) Gebauer Company.

www.nordstroms.com Nordstrom Department Store. Good selection of bras.

www.thebreastcancersite.com Information and merchandise.

Hospitals that specialize in BreastCancer Treatment

There are cancer centers and hospitals that specialize in breast cancer. Often information on clinical trials is more readily available at a larger hospital. You may find yourself going to one hospital for a primary treatment but receiving follow-up more locally. Again, insurance is a consideration and you should check with your insurance company to see if it will cover you out-of-state. Sometimes this may work to your advantage when out-of-state doctors and hospitals are providers in your insurance system. These are just some of the centers.

UCLA, Revlon Breast Center, Los Angeles, California
310-825-5268
M.D. Anderson, University of Texas, Houston, Texas
713-792-2121
Mayo Clinic, Rochester, Minnesota
507-284-3753
Johns Hopkins, Baltimore, Maryland
410-955-8822
Sloan-Kettering, New York, New York
212-639-2000
Duke University Medical Center, Durham, North Carolina
919-684-5613
City Of Hope, Duarte, California
626-256-4676
Dana-Farber/ Harvard Cancer Center, Boston, Massachusetts
617-632-2161
UCSF, San Francisco, California
415-502-1710

Questions to Ask Your Doctor

All these questions may not pertain to your case but they are questions that may help you organize your thoughts. It is your option to tear it out, copy it and take it to the doctor's office with you. Again, I suggest you take a friend or relative to accompany you to your appointments when possible.

Today's date:

Doctor's name:

Facility:

What and when was my last test?

What kind of breast cancer do I have?

What is the exact diagnosis?

How was this determined?

What stage is my cancer?

What makes it that stage?

I would like copies of my reports/films. How can that be arranged?

Has the cancer spread beyond my breast?

Is it in my lymph nodes or beyond?

How will you determine if that is the case?

Is it in more than one location in my breast?

Am I node negative or node positive?

What is my HER/2nue status?

Do I need more tests to determine if it has spread?

Do I need surgery?

Do you recommend a lumpectomy or mastectomy?

Will I be having a sentinel node biopsy?

How soon should I start treatment?

Do I need a second opinion?

What are my treatment options?

In what order do you suggest?

Do I need chemotherapy?

What kind of chemotherapy?

Where will this be done?

For how long and how often?

Do I need radiation?

Before or after surgery?

For how long?

Where will that take place?

Should I get a radiation boost?

Are there other options?

If my treatment includes chemotherapy, will I get a port?

What side effects can I expect?

Will I be able to work while I am being treated?

What are the real numbers as to how the treatment affects my survival and recurrence rates?

Do I need a plastic surgeon?

What are my plastic surgery options?

Whom do you recommend to do the surgery?

Do you have recommendations and their phone numbers?

Will it be just one surgery?

What are the possible complications?

How long will I be in the hospital?

Will I go home with a drain?

If I opt for reconstruction will it happen at the same time?

What are the side effects of surgery?

How much will it cost?

Do you take my insurance?

Do all the doctors involved take my insurance?

Is the anesthesiologist covered by my insurance?

Where will the surgery be done?

What kind of help do you think I will need while I am being treated?

Do I need radiation after surgery?

If so for how long?

What are the side effects?

What kind of follow-up do you recommend?

How often will I have to be tested in the future and what are the tests that you recommend?

What prescription medicine will I be on if any? What are the side effects? Explain if you are currently taking any medicine.

How will you know if you got it all?

What follow-up will I need?

Should I be genetically tested?

What do I need to do to get tested?

What does that cost?

What are the downsides of being tested?

What are the best things I can do to feel good again?

When I have my blood pressure taken or blood draws done in the future which arm should they use?

Also request that copies of all your reports be sent to your GP – general practitioner, your Ob-Gyn and/or anyone else on your care team. Have the fax numbers or email addresses available so you can give them to the doctor's office. And ask for a copy of the reports for you to read and keep.

Susan's "Love Dog" soup

A good easy-to-make soup to keep on hand as you are recovering.

1 onion
1 celery stalk
5 carrots
1 package of spinach (or one large can of spinach)
1 can of whole tomatoes
1 can of black beans (drained and rinsed)
Olive oil
32 oz of chicken stock
64 oz of water (more if you want more broth)
Salt and pepper to taste
Fresh basil if you have it
½ box of Orzo (or you could add other small pasta)
Grated cheese

You need a large soup pot with lid. Saute chopped onion in olive oil that coats bottom of pot over medium heat. Add chopped carrots and celery. Let cook for 5-10 minutes and stir. Add chicken stock, package of spinach, black beans and can of tomatoes. Add water, salt and pepper, chopped basil and orzo, turn up heat and bring to boil for 5 minutes. Turn off heat and let sit on stove for 15 minutes. Serve just made or refrigerate and put into bowls and top with grated cheese and microwave to re-heat.

www.ingramcontent.com/pod-product-compliance
Lightning Source LLC
LaVergne TN
LVHW091029080826
845145LV00002B/406

* 9 7 8 0 6 1 5 6 6 5 3 5 1 *